HEALTH FOR THE PACIFIC 5

Drugs of Addiction

in Papua New Guinea

by Richard Jones

AF583502

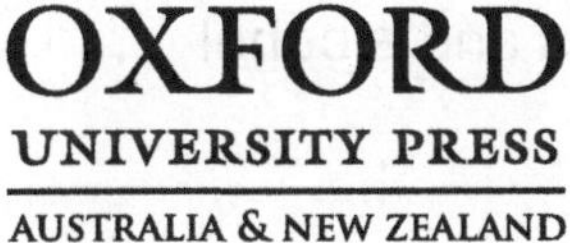
OXFORD
UNIVERSITY PRESS
AUSTRALIA & NEW ZEALAND

Contents

Foreword and acknowledgments iii

Notes for teachers iv

Introduction 1

Chapter 1 What are drugs? 2

Chapter 2 Medicines 6

Chapter 3 Why do people use drugs and alcohol? 10

Chapter 4 Alcohol 12

Chapter 5 Tobacco 23

Chapter 6 Betelnut 32

Chapter 7 Kava and caffeine 36

Chapter 8 Marijuana 38

Chapter 9 Petrol, glue, aerosols and amphetamines 43

Chapter 10 Illegal drugs in other countries 45

Chapter 11 Resisting drugs and alcohol 48

Chapter 12 Giving up drugs and alcohol 51

Chapter 13 HIV/AIDS 61

Summary of drugs of addiction 62

More information about drugs and alcohol 66

Glossary 67

Foreword

The lack of clear, simple and accurate information about good health contributes to poor health in any society.

This series is intended to educate and highlight important health issues that are affecting the lives of young men and women in the Pacific region.

The abuse of drugs and alcohol contribute to ill health so there is a need to educate our young people about these issues. They need to know the risks associated with drug and alcohol use, and the preventive measures that can reduce their impact in our communities, villages, towns and cities.

Health is everyone's concern.

Acknowledgments

Drug and alcohol abuse in Papua New Guinea is an important development issue and a serious concern for families, schools and communities. This booklet is designed to clearly present the facts about drugs and alcohol, and help develop the life skills of young men and women. Many young people are introduced to drugs and alcohol by their friends. It is important that they develop the skills to resist peer pressure.

The text is written to support the teaching of Personal Development in Papua New Guinea primary schools from Grade 6 onwards. It is a booklet for students and a resource book for teachers.

I would like to thank the many dedicated teachers and teacher trainers in the Department of Education who teach life skills to their students, and who help guide young people through the challenges in their life. I dedicate this book to them.

Richard Jones

Notes for teachers

This booklet has been written for Upper Primary and Lower Secondary school students studying the Personal Development subject. The knowledge, skills and attitudes developed in the text contribute to these learning outcomes from Personal Development:

Personal Development Grades 6–8

6.4.11 Describe the beneficial and harmful effects of drugs on health

6.4.12 Identify reasons people use drugs

7.4.11 Describe decisions people make about drug use and the result of those decisions on the community and individuals

7.4.12 Propose ways of responding to pressures to use harmful substances

8.4.11 Evaluate the effects of drug use on the community

8.4.12 Describe the programs offered by support agencies and counselling programs in the community

Personal Development Grades 9–10

9.3.1 Identify relevant health and hygiene issues in their community

9.3.3 Explain and demonstrate strategies in dealing with a relevant health issue safely

10.2.2 Identify characteristics of positive peer groups that contribute to class and school spirit.

There are also strong curriculum links with Social Science, Language and Making a Living.

There are many activities in the text for the students to complete and discuss. These can be used for self-study or as teaching and learning activities in class. They are designed to assist maximum student participation and the development of life skills.

Introduction

There are many challenges for young men and women growing up in our country. Drugs and alcohol are two of these important health issues.

Young people use drugs and alcohol for many reasons. Most young people are introduced to drugs and alcohol by their friends and through peer pressure.

Young people need to know the facts about drugs and alcohol, and they need to know how to make safe and careful decisions about using them. Using drugs and alcohol can put you and others at risk. Many communities and families have been badly affected by drug and alcohol abuse.

The knowledge and life skills you will learn from this book can help you keep yourself healthy and improve the health of your community.

Chapter 1 What are drugs?

A drug is a chemical substance that changes your body. The effects of drugs can be physical, mental or emotional.

Some drugs are legal and others are illegal. Some drugs are very common and others are only used by a few people. Some drugs have very strong effects. Some drugs can help your body and others can be harmful or lead to dangerous behaviour.

Legal drugs in Papua New Guinea

Legal drugs can include prescription or non-prescription medicines. There are also several legal drugs that are not medicines and can be bought or grown in the community – alcohol, tobacco, caffeine and kava. These drugs can also be abused and can lead to poor health and unsafe behaviour.

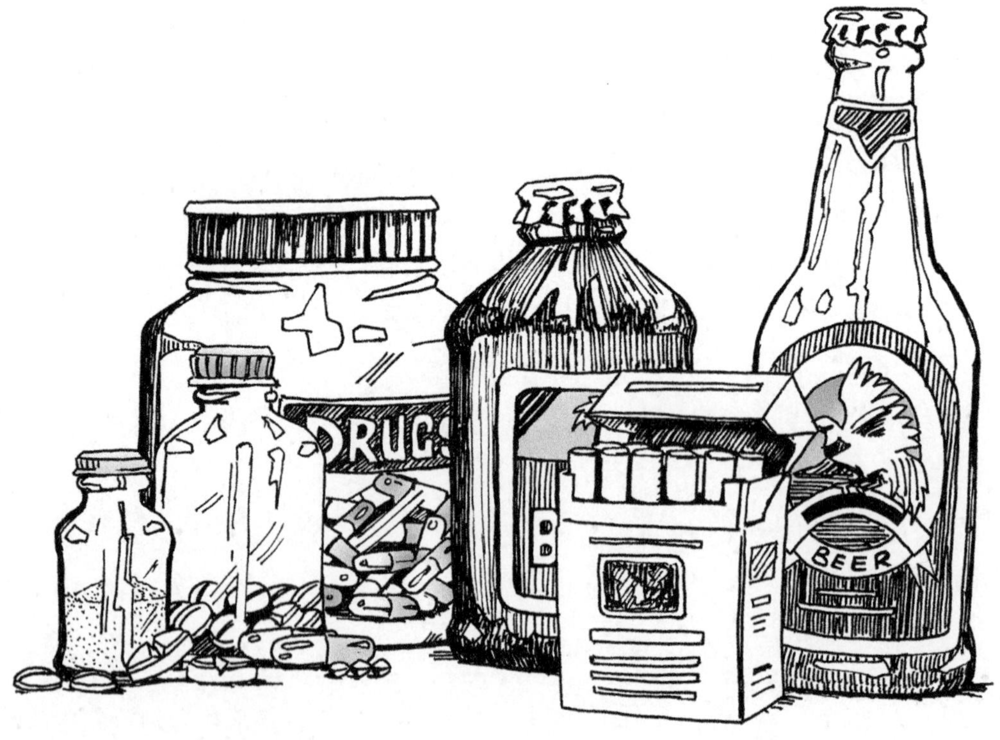

There are often laws about who can buy these drugs and when they can buy these drugs. If you understand and accept the risks, and you do not break the law, you can use them. Because these drugs are legal, many young people and adults use them. However, legal drugs have a huge impact on health in our country. Young men and women need to know how to say "no" to these drugs or use them safely and sensibly. Remember, all drugs change your body and there is a consequence for abusing them.

 Illegal drugs in Papua New Guinea

There are two main illegal drugs used in PNG – home-brew alcohol and marijuana. It is against the law to grow, make, transport, sell, buy or use these two drugs.

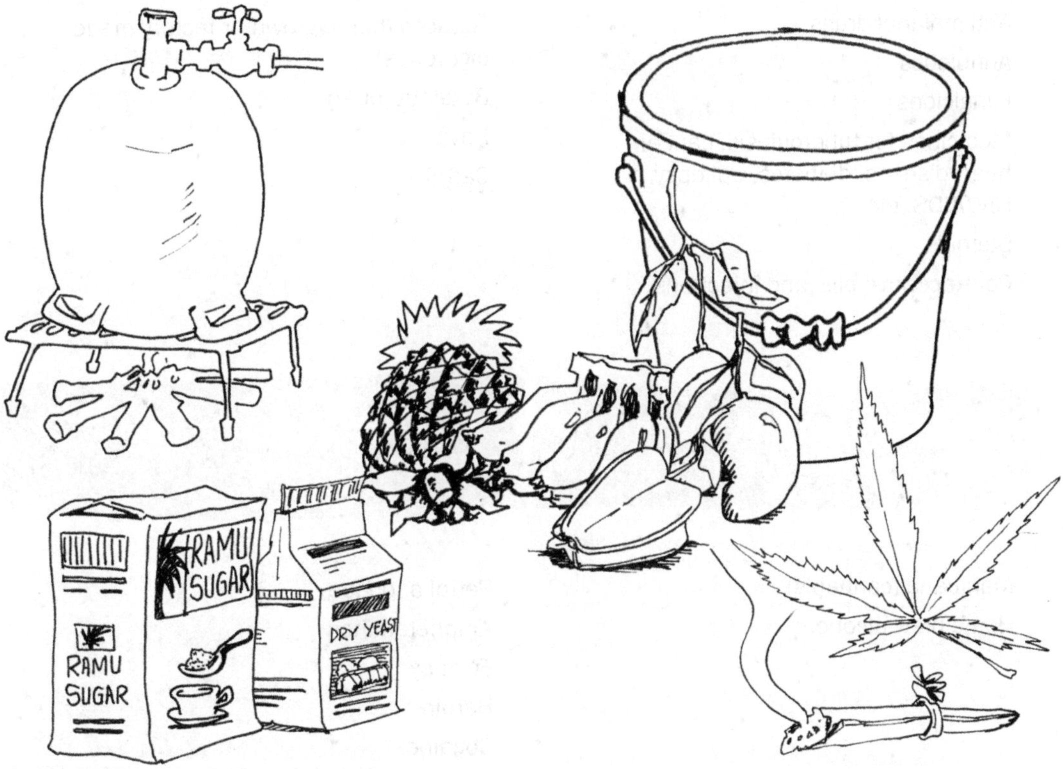

There are many serious health and criminal consequences for selling and using these illegal drugs. They can have a harmful impact on communities and young people. They might damage your health or lead to dangerous behaviour. These drugs are usually shared between friends and are widely available in markets or from street-sellers in cities, towns and villages. Some people make or grow these drugs for personal use or for sharing with their friends. Some people sell them.

LEGAL AND ILLEGAL DRUGS

Legal medicines	Legal drugs
Painkillers (paracetamol, etc.) Anti-malarial drugs Antibiotics Fungicides Medicines for tuberculosis, cancer, heart disease, diabetes, epilepsy, HIV/AIDS, etc. Steroids Contraceptive pills and injections	Alcohol Tobacco (home-grown or factory-made cigarettes) Betelnut (buai) Kava Caffeine
Common illegal drugs in Papua New Guinea	**Common illegal drugs in other countries**
Marijuana (cannabis) Home-brew alcohol	Petrol and glue Amphetamines Ecstasy Heroin Cocaine LSD (acid)

Activity 1·1

Work in groups to discuss drugs and answer the questions below:

1 Which drugs have you heard about in your community?
2 How do they affect people?
3 What do you think about when you hear the word "drugs"?
4 Check the drugs you talked about against the table on the previous page. Did you think of them all?

Facts about drugs and alcohol in PNG

- Ninety per cent of adults and young people have tried legal alcohol.
- The average age when they first tried alcohol is 16–17 years old.
- Sixty-four per cent of adults and young people have tried home-brew.
- The average age when they first tried drinking home-brew is 18–19 years old.
- Fifty-five per cent of adults and young people have tried smoking marijuana.
- The average age when they first tried smoking marijuana is 18 years old.
- Seventy per cent of males but only thirty per cent of females have tried marijuana.
- Ninety per cent of adults and young people have tried chewing betelnut.
- The average age when they first tried chewing betelnut is 12 years old.

Chapter 2 Medicines

Medicines are legal drugs that a health worker can give you if you are sick. There are many different medicines for treating illnesses. You can buy some of these from the pharmacy or collect them from the local health centre or hospital. Medicines can be in the form of pills, injections, liquids or creams. Some medicines are stronger and you need a prescription from a doctor or health worker to get them. In hospitals, doctors can prescribe strong medicines and painkillers for conditions such as HIV/AIDS, heart disease, tuberculosis or cancer.

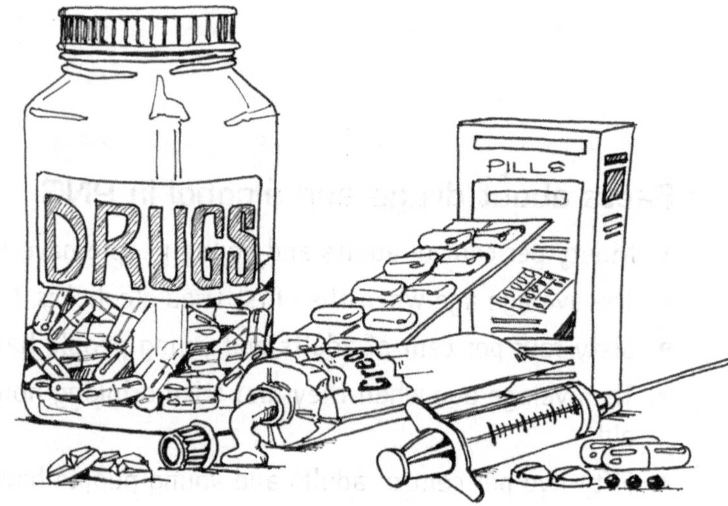

Activity 2·1

Work in groups to discuss medicines and answer the questions below:

1 Which medicines do you and your family take?
2 Where do you get them?
3 Which illnesses do they treat?
4 Are any of the medicines dangerous?
5 Which ones are prescription medicines?

Common medicines in PNG

Common medicines you can find in communities include:

- painkillers like paracetamol (Panadol) and aspirin
- antibiotics like amoxicillin and penicillin
- anti-malarial medicines like chloroquine, artemeter and Fansidar
- worming tablets
- grille and fungicide creams
- contraceptive pills and injections.

Using medicines safely

It is important that people taking medicines follow the instructions given by their doctor or health worker. Some medicines can damage your body if they are not taken correctly. Taking too much of a drug is called an overdose.

Sometimes medicines can have side effects. They should not be mixed with other medicines or alcohol. Always follow the instructions from the health worker and learn to read the labels on medicines. If you do not understand the instructions, ask a health worker or your pharmacist.

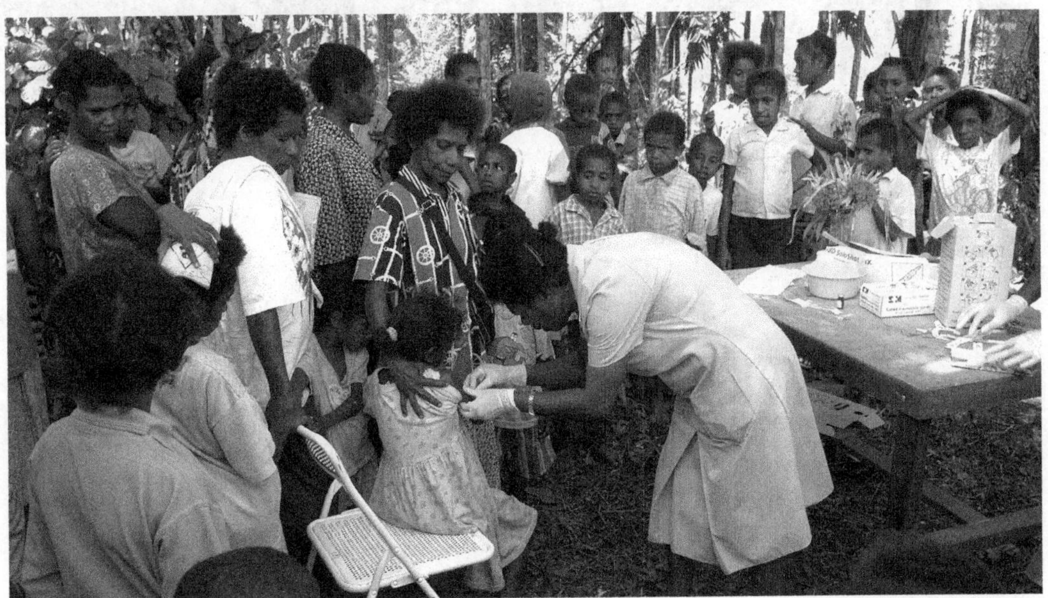

Buying medicines from markets is a serious health risk. These are usually drugs stolen from government health centres and warehouses. They are called black market medicines. This is a serious problem in PNG.

Another serious problem is when people do not finish their course of medicines. When they start to feel better they stop taking the medicine, but the germ that causes the illness is still in their body. The germ can become resistant to the medicine. This can be very dangerous the next time you or someone in your family gets sick. Malaria, HIV and tuberculosis are all diseases that are becoming resistant to medicines, so doctors find it harder to treat them and need to develop stronger medicines.

Some people abuse legal medicines and seriously damage their body; for example, taking steroids for bodybuilding or taking an overdose of painkillers.

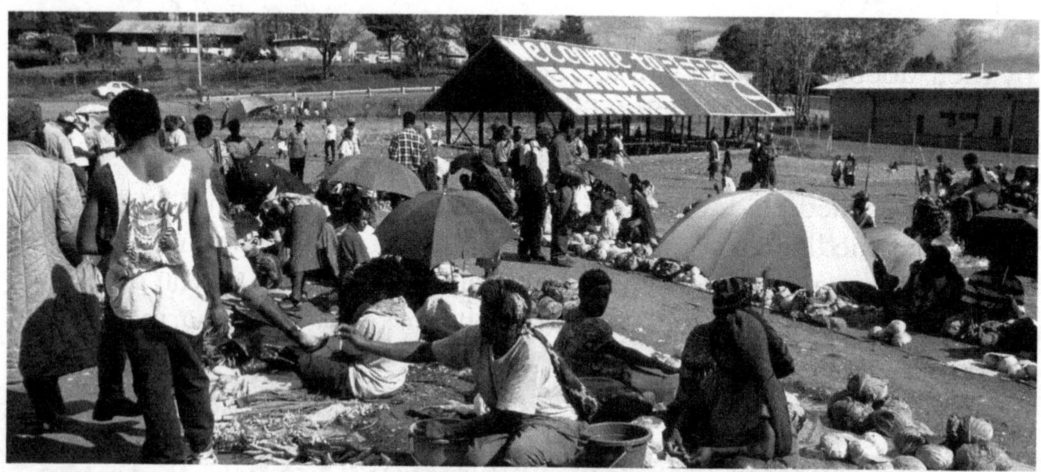

Activity 2·2

1 Which medicines can you buy in your local market?
2 Does anyone from your family or community buy medicines from the market? Why?

The risks of black market medicines

- they might be stolen
- they might be out of date
- they could be fakes
- you might not get the right dose
- you might be giving money to criminals.

Traditional medicines

Many people use traditional medicines and herbs to treat their illnesses. These medicines can be made from plants, animals and insects. Many of them are a very important part of traditional life.

Some traditional medicines may work but few have been scientifically tested. Some might not work at all and some might even be dangerous. For example, people sell herbs that they say can cure serious illnesses like HIV/AIDS or cancer. There is no evidence that these herbs can cure serious diseases. Vulnerable and desperate people pay a lot of money for these herbs but they do not work.

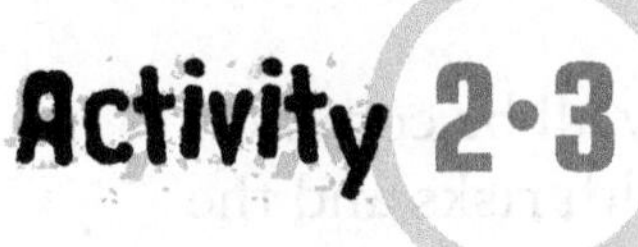

Sit down with a friend and interview an old person from your community about traditional medicines.

1 Which diseases and illnesses were they used to treat?

2 Are any of them still used today in your community?

Chapter 3 Why do people use drugs and alcohol?

Common reasons young people give for using drugs and alcohol include:

- experimenting
- wanting to feel good or feel high
- curiosity
- peer pressure – not wanting to be left out or look scared
- wanting to escape from a problem
- boredom
- traditional ceremonies
- social gathering to make people feel good
- sharing culture
- being part of cult or peer activity in school
- being tricked into it
- trying to look older and clever to increase their social status
- copying parents, siblings or role models who use them
- not knowing the health risks.

Some drugs are legal and some are not but they may all be common in your community. You need to understand the health risks and the consequences of abusing these drugs. Many people don't use drugs or are able to stop using them. They learn to resist the pressure to use drugs. You can make this choice too.

Why use alcohol and tobacco?

'My school mates and my older brothers all smoked cigarettes and I was curious about how it felt. It was pretty exciting the first time.' **Dipa**

'When I have had a difficult day I need to escape. I like to have a beer and relax. It's good for me. I buy beers for my mates and look like a bikman.' **Samuel**

'Smoking spak brus (marijuana) makes me laugh and feel good. I only smoke it sometimes when I need to be confident. We always smoke in the gang after school. It's exciting.' **Bobbi**

'I started chewing when I was really young and now I have a chew every day. I don't chew at work but I normally have three or four buai a day. Besides, everyone in PNG chews, don't they?' **Ana**

'All my mates drink home-brew out in the gardens. Life in the village is so boring. I don't want to be the odd one out so I drink too, but I try not to get into trouble.' **John**

'Sharing your cigarettes with your friends is cool and the right thing to do. We look older, I think. And anyway, everyone smokes in my class.' **Elisabeth**

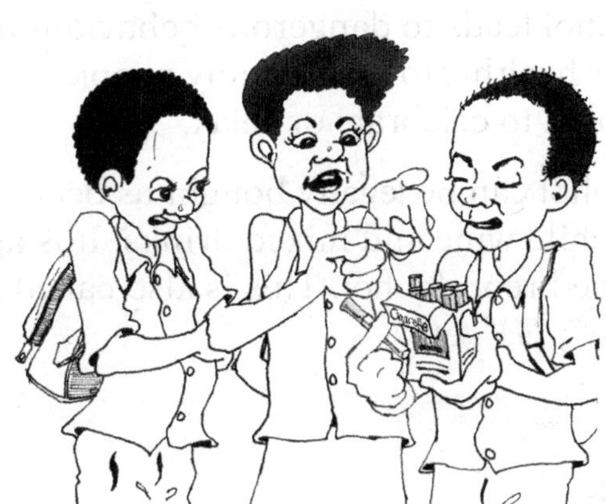

Activity 3·1

1 Why do these people use drugs or alcohol? List the reasons.
2 Which reasons are common for drug and alcohol use in your community? Why?
3 What other reasons are there for using drugs and alcohol? (For example, traditional ceremonies.)

Chapter 4 Alcohol

Alcohol is the most common legal drug in our country. It is also the one that causes the most problems in families and communities. Abusing alcohol leads to dangerous behaviour and violence and can damage your health. However, many people drink safely and responsibly and use alcohol to celebrate or relax.

Alcohol can be legally bought as beer, spirits (like whisky or vodka), red or white wine and mixed drinks. It is against the law to make your own home-brew alcohol. This is also called "jungle juice", "yawa", "home-brew", "JJ", etc.

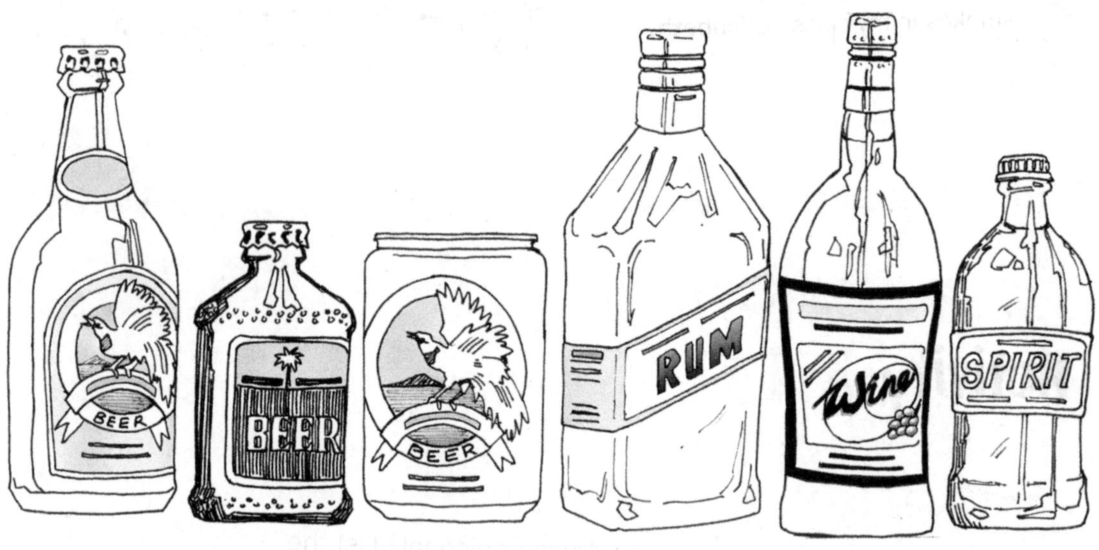

Facts about alcohol

- Alcohol is a chemical called ethanol.
- Alcoholic drinks are a mix of ethanol with water and other flavours.
- Alcohol is made from sugar by a microbe called yeast.
- People have been brewing alcohol for thousands of years.
- Your body must break down the alcohol because it is a poison.
- Your body does this in the liver.
- Alcohol changes your behaviour.
- The effects of alcohol depend on your gender, your body size and how fast you drink.

Laws about alcohol

- You have to be at least 18 to buy alcohol.
- It is against the law to drive a car if you have been drinking.
- It is against the law to buy alcohol for someone younger than 18.
- Some provinces and communities are "dry" – alcohol is banned there.
- It is against the law to brew your own alcohol.

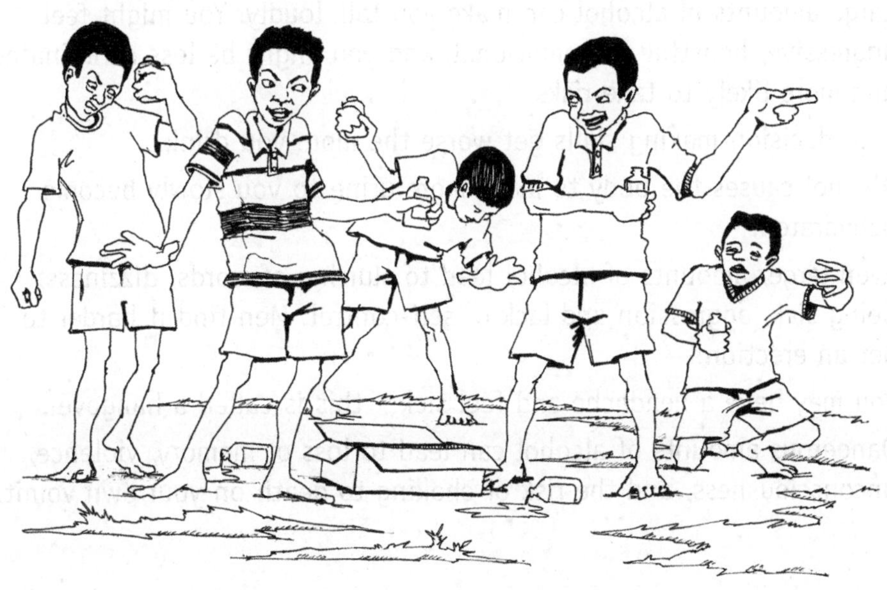

How does alcohol affect the body?

1 Small amounts of alcohol may make you feel lively, cheerful and confident.

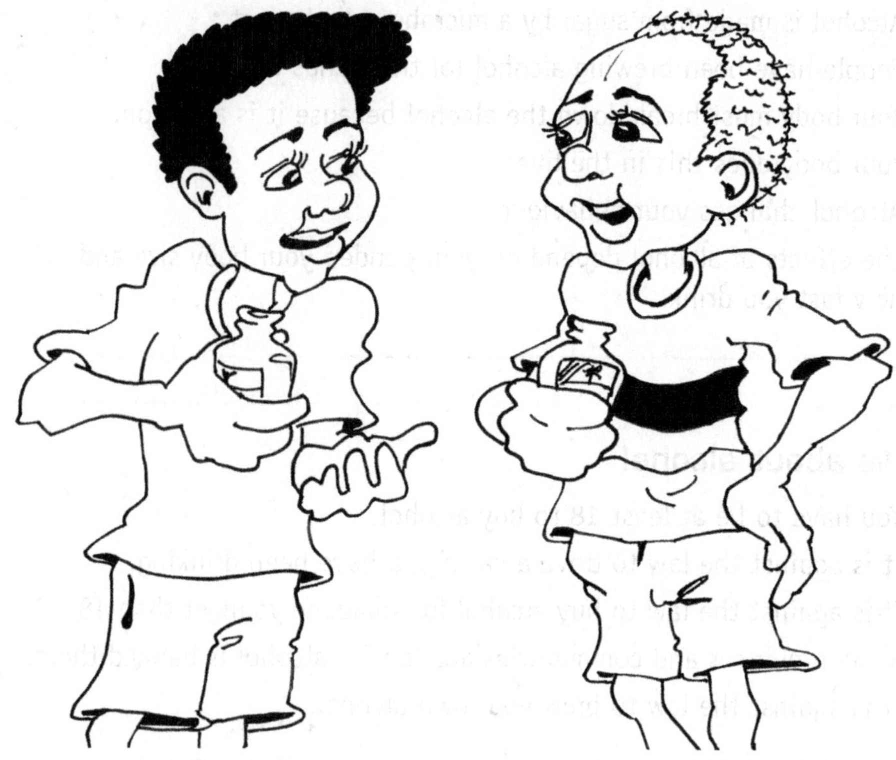

2 Large amounts of alcohol can make you talk loudly. You might feel aggressive, boastful and emotional, and you might be less coordinated and more likely to take risks.

3 Your decision-making skills get worse the more you drink.

4 Alcohol causes the body to make more urine so you slowly become dehydrated.

5 Even larger amounts of alcohol lead to slurring of words, dizziness, being sick, aggression and lack of self-control. Men find it harder to get an erection.

6 You may have a headache and feel sick – this is called a hangover.

7 Dangerous amounts of alcohol can lead to loss of memory, violence, unconsciousness, and the risk of choking to death on your own vomit.

Alcohol and your health

There are many risks from abusing alcohol. Alcohol is addictive and some people find they cannot stop drinking and getting drunk. This is called alcoholism. People who drink too much or "binge-drink" (get drunk or "six-to-six") have many health and behaviour problems.

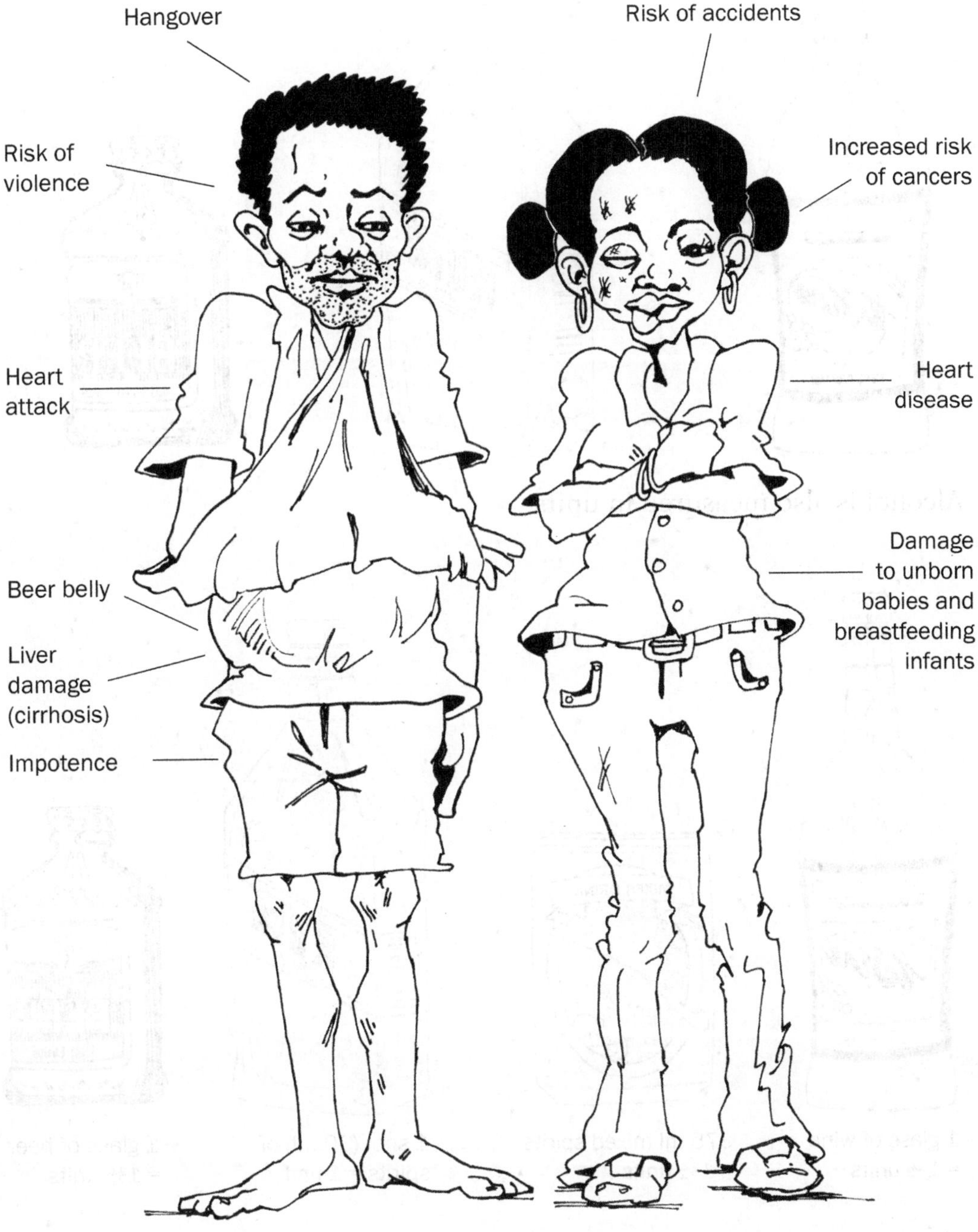

Hangover
Risk of accidents
Risk of violence
Increased risk of cancers
Heart attack
Heart disease
Beer belly
Damage to unborn babies and breastfeeding infants
Liver damage (cirrhosis)
Impotence

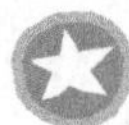

Safe drinking limits

The strength of the alcohol in bottles is written on the label: the higher the percentage of alcohol, the stronger the alcoholic drink.

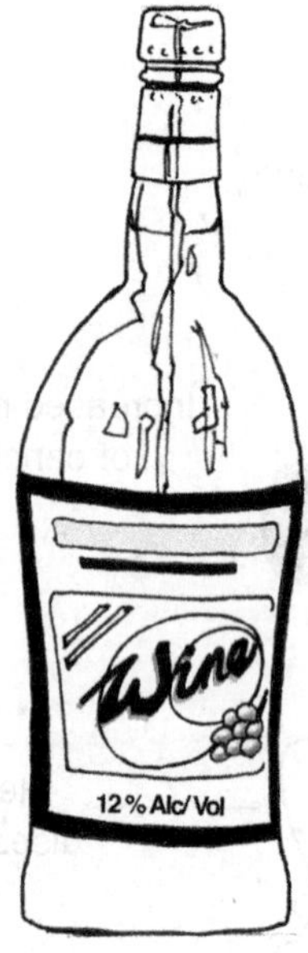

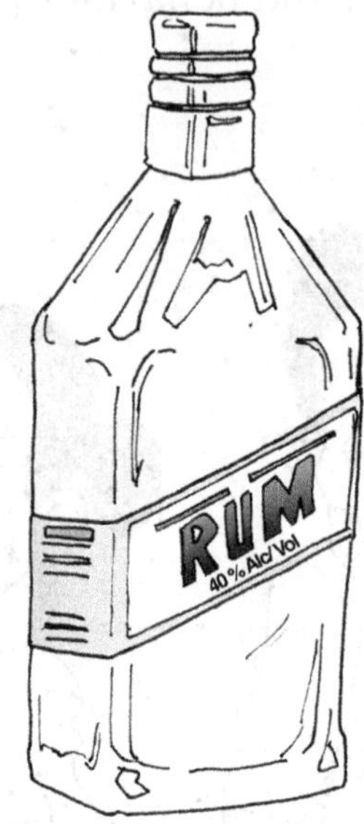

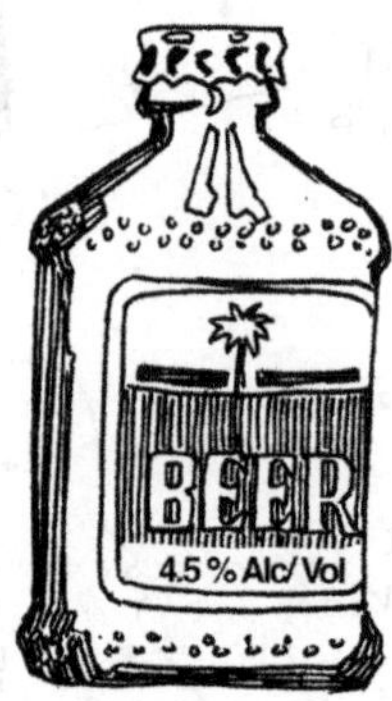

Alcohol is also measured in units.

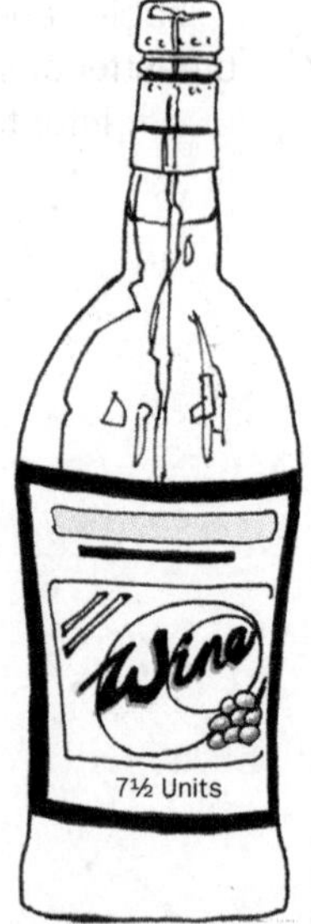

1 glass of wine = 1½ units

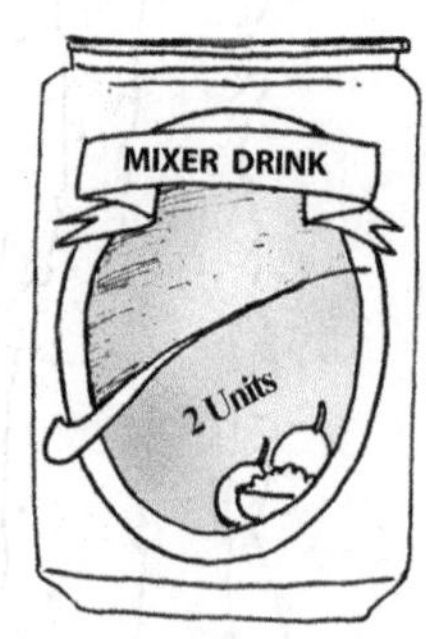

375 ml mixed spirits = 1½ units

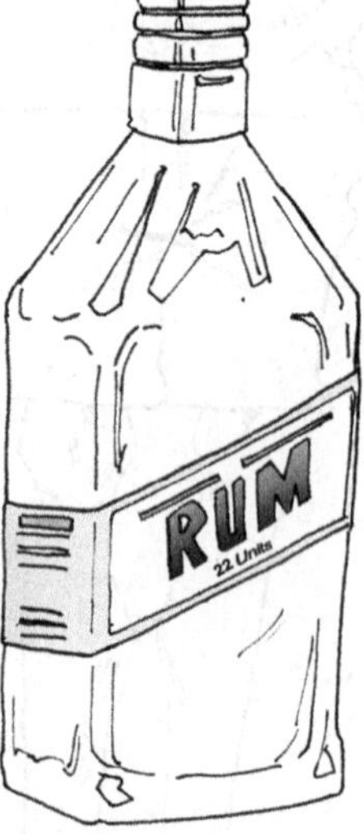

1 shot (30 ml) of spirits = 1 unit

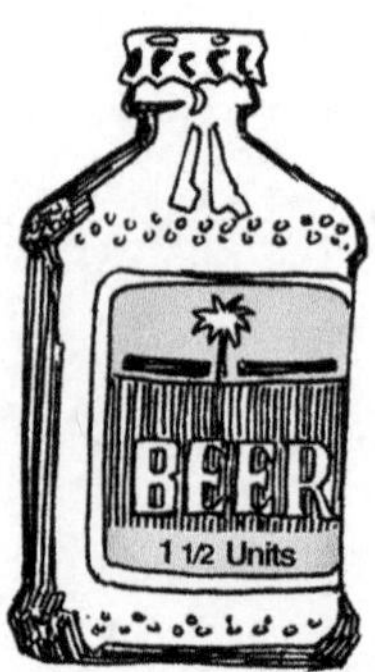

1 glass of beer = 1½ units

The Department of Health recommends the maximum safe amount of alcohol a person can drink each week without experiencing serious health effects. A man can drink a maximum of 21 units a week (or 4 units a day) and a woman can drink a maximum of 14 units a week (or 3 units a day). Pregnant and breastfeeding women should not drink at all. The more you drink above the safe limits, the more harmful alcohol is likely to be.

Remember, binge-drinking can be harmful even though the weekly total may not seem too high. And you can't tell the strength of home-brew alcohol – this is one of the reasons it is so dangerous.

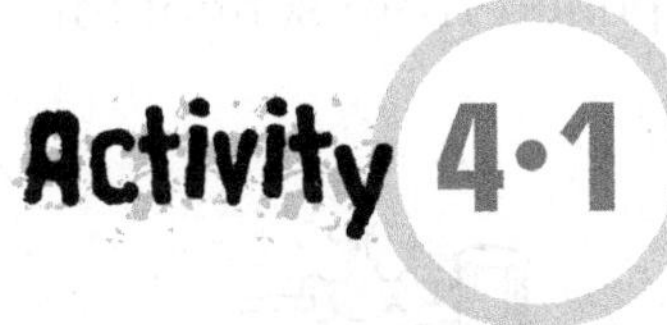

- Read these diaries and calculate how many units of alcohol George and Cathy drink in a week. Do you think they have a health problem? Why?

George

Monday: three bottles of beer

Tuesday: nothing

Wednesday: six-pack of beer

Thursday: bottle of wine

Friday: three vodkas and three beers

Saturday: one beer while watching TV

Cathy

Monday: nothing

Tuesday: three mixer drinks with friends

Wednesday: nothing

Thursday: two glasses of wine

Friday: three vodka mixers

Saturday: two glasses of wine, two beers

Home-brew

Home-brew is alcohol made from sugar, yeast and mashed-up fruit. This mixture is left to ferment and then it is distilled to collect the alcohol. The alcohol is very strong so it is usually mixed with cordial for drinking. Making home-brew is illegal in PNG.

Home-brew is very dangerous. If it is not distilled carefully it can be poisonous and lead to blindness or death. Because home-brew is very strong, drinking it can quickly lead to drunkenness, fights and risky behaviour. Many communities ban home-brew and police will destroy any home-brew equipment they find. You can be expelled from school for making or drinking home-brew.

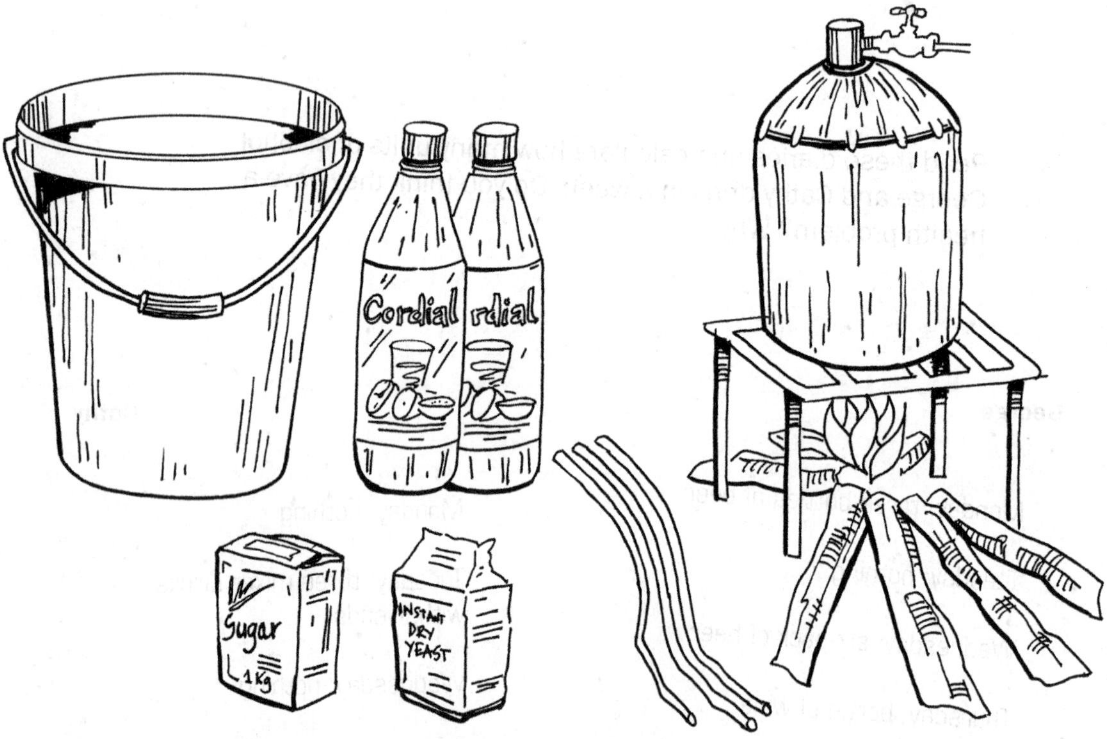

Alcohol abuse and the community

The abuse of alcohol is probably the most serious addiction facing PNG. It is a particular problem for many men. Some men drink all night until they have lost all self-control. This binge-drinking leads to many problems including violence. This is alcohol abuse.

Activity 4·2

1 With a partner, discuss people in your community who make and drink home-brew. You can use false names. List the reasons why they make and drink home-brew.

2 Decide which reasons you will use to say "no" to home-brew.

3 List the consequences of making and drinking home-brew (in school, in the community and in your family).

4 List the risks for young men and women from drinking alcohol. Are the risks the same? What are the gender differences?

EFFECTS OF ALCOHOL ABUSE

The individual	The family	The community
• Wasted money • Health damage • Possible addiction • Leads to risk-taking behaviour like unprotected sex • Could lead to violence and rape	• Domestic violence and rape • Wasting money that could be spent on school fees or daily living • Could lead to unfaithfulness and family breakdown	• Making home-brew is against the law • Damage to property • Jealousy and arguments • Noise and disturbance at night • Compensation for drunken behaviour • Wastes resources • Drunk drivers kill or injure innocent people

Daniel's story

Daniel's father likes to drink. Every pay Friday, he stays out late with his mates in the local bar. He comes home late at night smelling of alcohol. Sometimes he is happy and brings food and rice. But sometimes he is short-tempered and throws things around the house. When he is drunk, he hits Daniel's mum and shouts at Daniel and his brothers and sisters. No one in the family or the community can seem to do anything about it. The next morning, Daniel's dad has a hangover and says sorry.

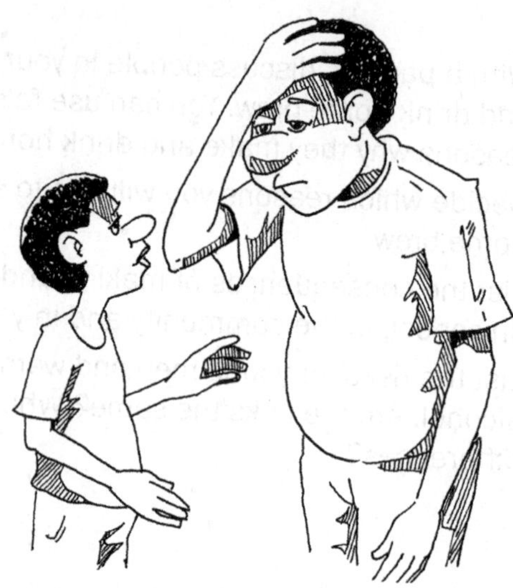

Activity 4·3

1 What are the effects of Daniel's dad's alcohol abuse?
2 How do you think Daniel, his mother and his father feel?
3 What are the causes of the violence in the house?
4 What should the family do?
5 What should the community do?
6 What might happen to Daniel's family in the future?

How do you know if you are addicted to alcohol?

If you stop drinking alcohol for a day or so, and you suffer unpleasant withdrawal symptoms, then you could be addicted to alcohol. For example, you feel sick, tremble, sweat and want alcohol. Some people end up drinking alcohol every day to avoid these symptoms.

Many men and some women drink too much. They might not be addicted to alcohol but it is still damaging their health.

How do you drink responsibly?

Some people do not drink alcohol at all. Some people can drink responsibly. They have self-control and behave sensibly. They don't get drunk or violent. How do they do this?

Responsible drinking

- Know when enough is enough.
- Don't drink to get drunk.
- Know how to resist peer pressure.
- Decide how many drinks you will have before you start drinking.
- Think about the consequences of drinking too much.
- Don't drink with friends who might get into trouble or do something risky or stupid.
- Drink slowly and alternate your alcoholic drinks with soft drinks and water.

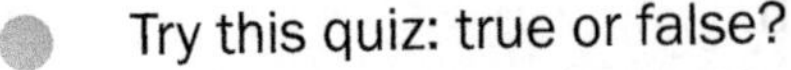

Activity 4·4

Try this quiz: true or false?

1 Drinking lots of water before going to sleep prevents any health damage from alcohol.
2 Drinking alcohol makes you more alert and energetic.
3 After a night of sleep, all the alcohol is gone from your body.
4 Drinking just over the recommended limits is not too harmful.
5 Coffee or betelnut will sober you up.
6 You shouldn't say "no" if someone offers you a drink.

The answers!

1 False! It might reduce the hangover but won't protect your liver from damage.
2 False! Alcohol might make you feel sharper but it actually slows your reactions down. It is a depressant.
3 False! Your body takes about one hour to break down one unit of alcohol. You can still be drunk when you wake up.
4 False! For example, if a man drinks five units each day he doubles his risk of developing liver disease, high blood pressure, cancer, and of having a violent death.
5 False! They might make you more alert but they won't remove the alcohol from your blood.
6 False! Although it is hard to say "no" when someone offers you a drink, you need to think about your own health.

Chapter 5 Tobacco

Tobacco is a legal drug that is common all over the world. It is made from the dried leaves of the tobacco plant. It contains many different chemicals but the one that makes it addictive is called nicotine. Nicotine is a powerful drug and it is very addictive.

Tobacco is one of the more dangerous drugs because of the long-term health damage smoking does to the body. Tobacco has killed millions of people. There will be people in your community who are ill because they smoke. On average, smokers have shorter lives than non-smokers.

In the Pacific region, people smoke tobacco in factory-made cigarettes or they roll their own cigarettes with dry tobacco and newspaper. Some people smoke tobacco in pipes. People who cannot afford a whole packet of cigarettes sometimes buy one "stick" from a market stall.

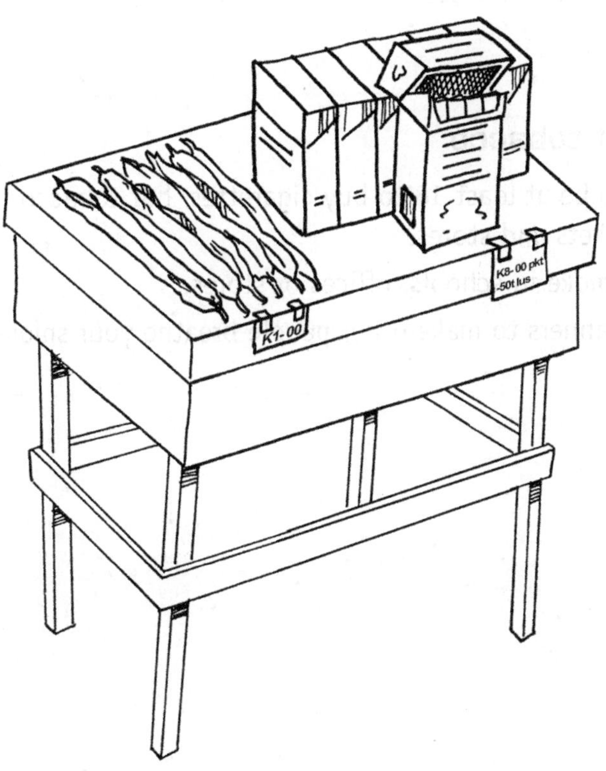

Many young people and children start smoking at an early age. They don't think it is doing them any harm but it is very hard to give up. Illnesses and damage from smoking will affect their health later in life. It is better never to smoke at all.

Facts about tobacco

- Smoke from tobacco contains many poisonous chemicals.
- Many of the chemicals in tobacco smoke are very poisonous and lead to heart disease, lung, throat and mouth cancers, breathing problems and serious ill health.
- Cigarettes contain tar, which is a black sticky liquid that stains your fingers, damages your throat and causes cancer.
- Factory-made cigarettes have a filter that removes a little of the tar, but this does not make the cigarettes less addictive or dangerous.
- The nicotine in cigarettes is so addictive that people's bodies soon want to have more – giving up smoking tobacco is very difficult because the body misses the nicotine.

Laws about tobacco

- You have to be at least 18 to buy cigarettes, but tobacco is widely sold in markets and stores.
- You can't smoke in schools, offices or stores.
- It is bad manners to make other people breathe your smoke.

Tobacco and your health

The serious health risks of smoking are well proven. Even if you only smoke a few times a day, the smoke is attacking the cells in your body. Half of all regular smokers die of smoking-related diseases and their life expectancy is 13 to 16 years less than that of non-smokers.

People who smoke regularly are not as fit as non-smokers because the smoke damages their lungs and blood. They easily get out of breath and the poisons in the smoke damage their throat and cause heart disease. People who smoke for many years have a much greater risk of cancer because of the damage to the cells in their body. Lung, throat and mouth cancers kill thousands of long-term smokers every year.

Smokers often have bad breath and smelly clothes too.

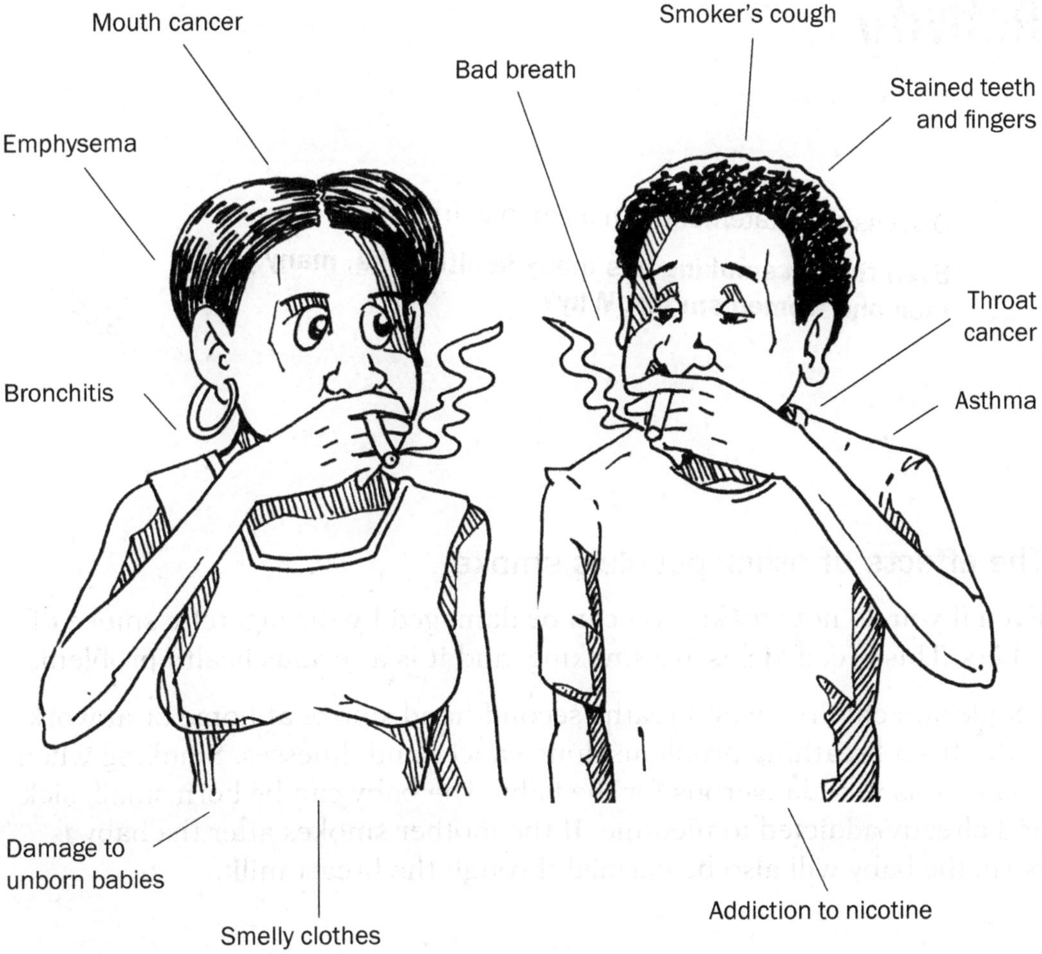

Mouth cancer
Smoker's cough
Bad breath
Stained teeth and fingers
Emphysema
Throat cancer
Bronchitis
Asthma
Damage to unborn babies
Smelly clothes
Addiction to nicotine

Gruesome smoking facts

Toxic chemicals in tobacco smoke include:

- nicotine – the addictive agent in tobacco smoke
- formaldehyde – used in preservation of laboratory specimens
- ammonia – used in toilet cleaner
- hydrogen cyanide – used in rat poison
- carbon monoxide - found in car exhaust
- tar – the black sticky liquid found on roads.

Discuss this statement with a group of friends:

Even though smoking has many health risks, many young men and women smoke. Why?

The effects of other people's smoke

Even if you do not smoke, you can be damaged by the cigarette smoke of others. This is called passive smoking, and it is a serious health problem.

People and children who breathe second-hand smoke at home or at work suffer from breathing problems, lung cancer and illnesses. Smoking when pregnant is very dangerous for the baby. The baby can be born small, sick and already addicted to nicotine. If the mother smokes after the baby is born, the baby will also be harmed through the breast milk.

Smoking in developing countries

In developed countries like the United States of America and Australia, there are many laws about smoking. You can't smoke inside a public building or workplace. Cigarette packets have pictures of dying people and damaged lungs and strong anti-smoking messages on them. There are campaigns to stop young people smoking and getting addicted to nicotine. Lawsuits have been filed against the cigarette companies for compensation, and cigarettes are taxed very heavily to make it harder for people to smoke.

In developing countries like PNG or the Solomon Islands, tobacco is cheap and widely available. Many people grow tobacco. There are no strict laws and many people are not aware of the huge risks of smoking. In fact, smoking kills and makes more people sick in developing countries than in developed ones. It is a serious health problem in the Pacific region.

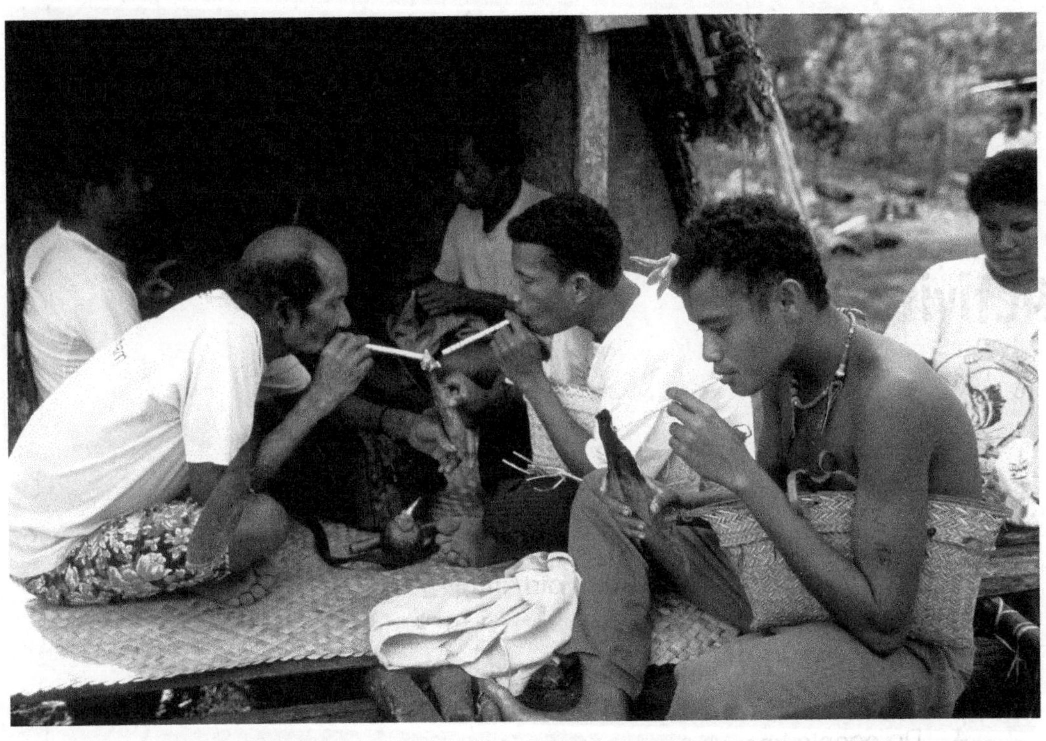

Activity 5·2

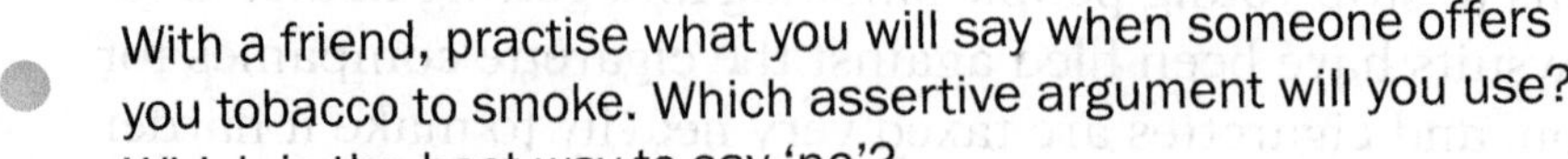

With a friend, practise what you will say when someone offers you tobacco to smoke. Which assertive argument will you use? Which is the best way to say 'no'?

Role-play what someone might say to persuade you to smoke and how you would say no. Try to be assertive, practise strong body language and use good reasons.
For example:

Terry: Bro, your turn.

Cornelius: No, mi les. I don't want to get started. Let's go and play some volleyball.

Activity 5·3

Survey different age groups to investigate what percentage of people in your community smoke.

1 Do more young people than old smoke?
2 Do more women than men?
3 What is the average number of 'sticks' people smoke in a day?
4 Do people know how smoking damages their health?

The effects of smoking on family and community

'When my papa smokes he wastes the money we should be spending on school fees. He also smells bad and I don't like breathing in the smoke.' **Jenny**

'My family makes good money from selling dry tobacco in the market which we use to pay for rice and tinned fish.' **Kena**

'We all stopped smoking when our baby was born. The smoke made her asthma worse and it was costing us a lot of money in medicine.' **Maria**

'Our neighbour's house burnt down when they were at the market. Someone told me they had left a cigarette burning when they left the house. It was very scary.' **Jimi**

'We don't let them sell cigarettes in the village store and our young people are much healthier and fitter. Hopefully we will have fewer sick people in years to come and our children won't be tempted to smoke. There is less litter too.' **Susie**

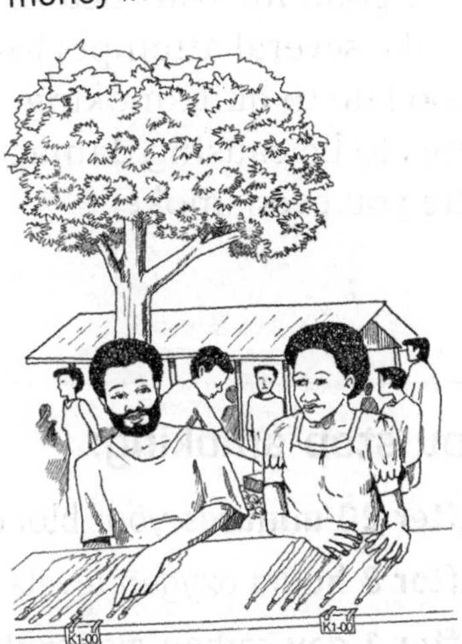

Activity 5·4

1. List the impacts of smoking on families.
2. List the impacts of smoking on communities.
3. List the ways that people try and prevent these problems.

 Giving up tobacco

If you stop smoking tobacco, your lungs start to recover almost straight away. You might cough more at the beginning as your body tries to remove the tar. But if you have bronchitis and asthma, these illnesses will start to get better. You will feel fitter, and reduce your risk of blood clots and heart disease. In time, your body will recover completely and your risk of getting cancer will be the same as a non-smoker.

Giving up smoking is very hard because nicotine is so addictive. Smokers still want to smoke because their body misses the nicotine. But giving up is very good for your health so many people try break their addiction. It may take several attempts to give up, but it is worth the effort. It is never too late to quit smoking. At the same time, it is never too early for cigarettes to be causing damage. Health damage begins with the first cigarette you ever smoke.

If you stop smoking:

- **After 20 minutes** your blood pressure and pulse return to normal.
- **After 8 hours** oxygen levels in your blood return to normal.
- **After 1 day** carbon monoxide is eliminated from the body and your lungs start to clear out mucus.
- **After 2 days** all the nicotine is gone from your body and your senses of taste and smell improve.
- **After 2 to 12 weeks** breathing becomes easier and you feel more energetic.
- **After 3 to 9 months** coughs, wheezes and breathing problems improve.
- **After 1 year** your risk of a heart attack falls to half that of a smoker.
- **After 10 years** your risk of lung cancer falls to half that of a smoker.
- **After 15 years** your risk of a heart attack falls to that of a non-smoker.

Getting started

- Tell your friends and family you are giving up and ask them to help.
- Set a date for giving up and stick to it.
- Keep a record of when you last smoked and how much money you have saved by not smoking.
- Practise how to say 'no' if someone offers you a cigarette.
- Chew sugar-free gum or keep some fruit handy to keep your mouth busy.
- Keep yourself busy with sport, reading, school work or community activities.
- Stay away from people and places where you might be tempted to have a cigarette.
- Don't replace one bad habit with another – if you give up smoking, don't chew more betelnut.
- Remind yourself of the health benefits of not smoking – your body is important, so look after it.
- Keep yourself active.

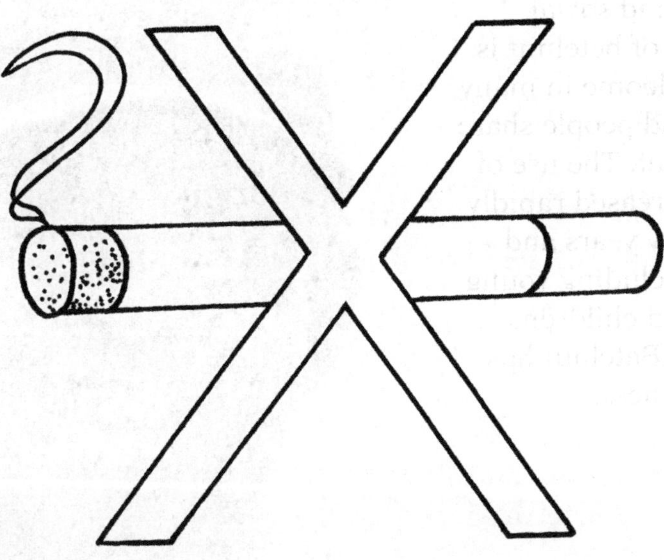

Chapter 6 Betelnut

Betelnut or *buai* is a legal drug that grows naturally in the Pacific region. It is a soft nut with a tough green skin. People chew the nut to feel a mild high. In some countries, they mix the chewed nut with powdered lime and mustard (*daka*).

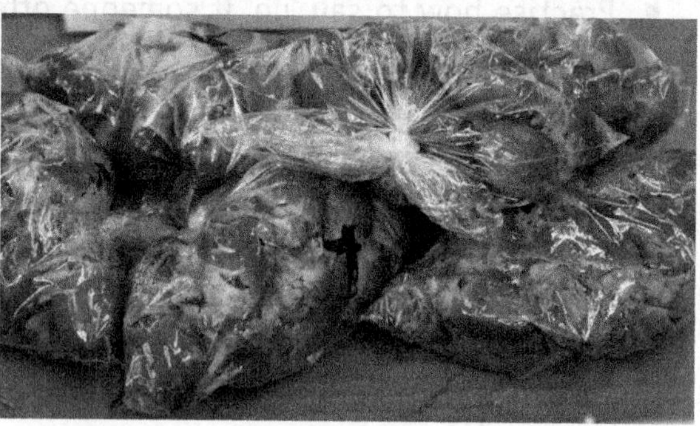

Betelnut is a traditional drug in many communities and it is widely used. However, chewing betelnut (especially with lime) damages the mouth and teeth and can lead to mouth cancer. It also produces lots of ugly red spit that spoils our environment and contributes to the spread of diseases like tuberculosis.

Betelnut is important in many cultural events and social meetings. A gift of betelnut is a traditional welcome in many communities and people share it when they meet. The use of betelnut has increased rapidly in the last twenty years and many people, including young men, women and children, chew every day. Betelnut has become big business.

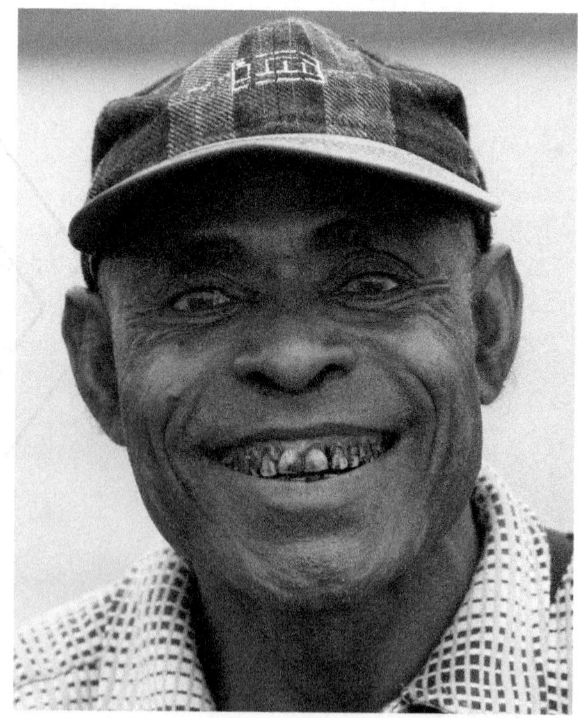

Facts about betelnut

- When betelnut is chewed, chemicals from the nut are absorbed into the body.
- Betelnut is addictive – the effects can last up to half an hour.
- Betelnut makes people feel alert, hot and sweaty, and reduces hunger pangs.
- Betelnut tastes very bitter and makes the body produce lots of saliva.
- Chewing betelnut increases the risk of mouth and throat cancers.
- Chewing betelnut with lime increases the damage to the mouth and can lead to sores, ulcers, cancers and badly stained and rotting teeth.

Laws about betelnut

- There are no laws about buying betelnut but some communities don't allow children to chew it.
- In towns, you can be fined for throwing betelnut shells and spitting in public.
- You are not allowed to chew betelnut in schools, stores or many workplaces.

Activity 6•1

Chewing betelnut is traditional in some communities. Research the use of betelnut in your community.

1 What is it used for?
2 What are the traditions about chewing?
3 Did people chew betelnut in the past?

How do you know if you are addicted to betelnut?

Betelnut is addictive and chewing it is a health risk. The signs of being addicted are:

- needing to chew in the morning when you get up
- stained teeth
- chewing every day
- chewing many times a day
- always offering or asking for betelnut, lime or mustard when you meet someone
- spending your money on betelnut, lime or mustard.

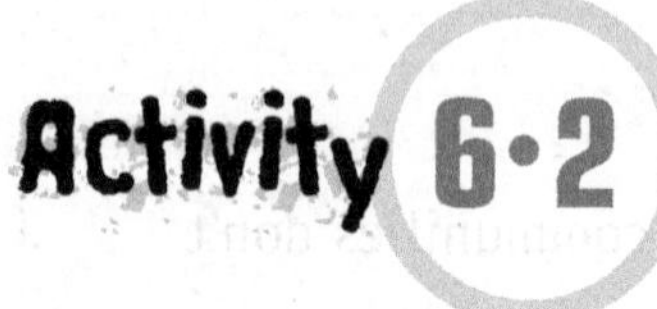

Your friend Helen is a serious betelnut chewer. You want to help her give up. What strategies would you and Helen use to help her reduce her chewing and eventually give up? (For example, is it cool to kiss a red stained mouth?)

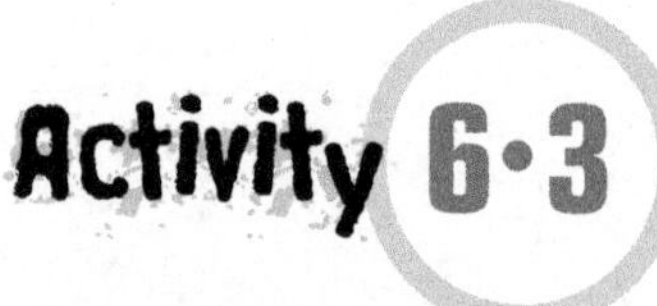

With a group of friends, discuss whether betelnut should be banned or not. What are the advantages and disadvantages of growing, selling, buying and using buai? List your recommendations for your community leaders.

The effects of betelnut:

- mild happiness and reduced hunger
- traditional social obligations and greetings
- sharing with others increases your social status
- making money in the informal sector or transporting betelnut
- increased risk of mouth and throat cancers
- stains on clothes, teeth and ground
- wastes money
- medical costs for cancer and damaged teeth
- littering and problems caused by informal stalls
- spitting spreads diseases like tuberculosis
- children start chewing because they see parents and older siblings using betelnut.

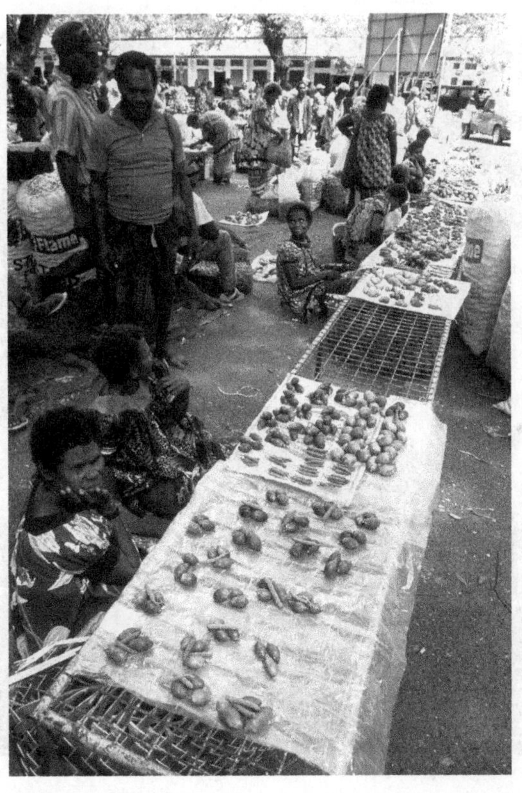

Chapter 7 Kava and caffeine

Kava is a legal natural drug used widely in some Pacific island countries. It is made from a special plant root. It is used to relieve stress and as an alternative to alcohol in social gatherings.

The kava root is ground up, mixed with water and carefully squeezed through a cloth to make a bitter, woody drink that numbs the mouth. It is a relaxant and the effects last a few hours depending on how strong the drink is made. It can make you sleepy and less likely to want to do work.

Kava is not addictive but people can get into the habit of drinking it. The health risks of kava are not yet clear. Drinking kava frequently may damage the liver and cause skin damage. Drinking kava for the first time, or drinking too quickly, can make you feel sick. It has a very bitter taste. Kava should not be mixed with alcohol.

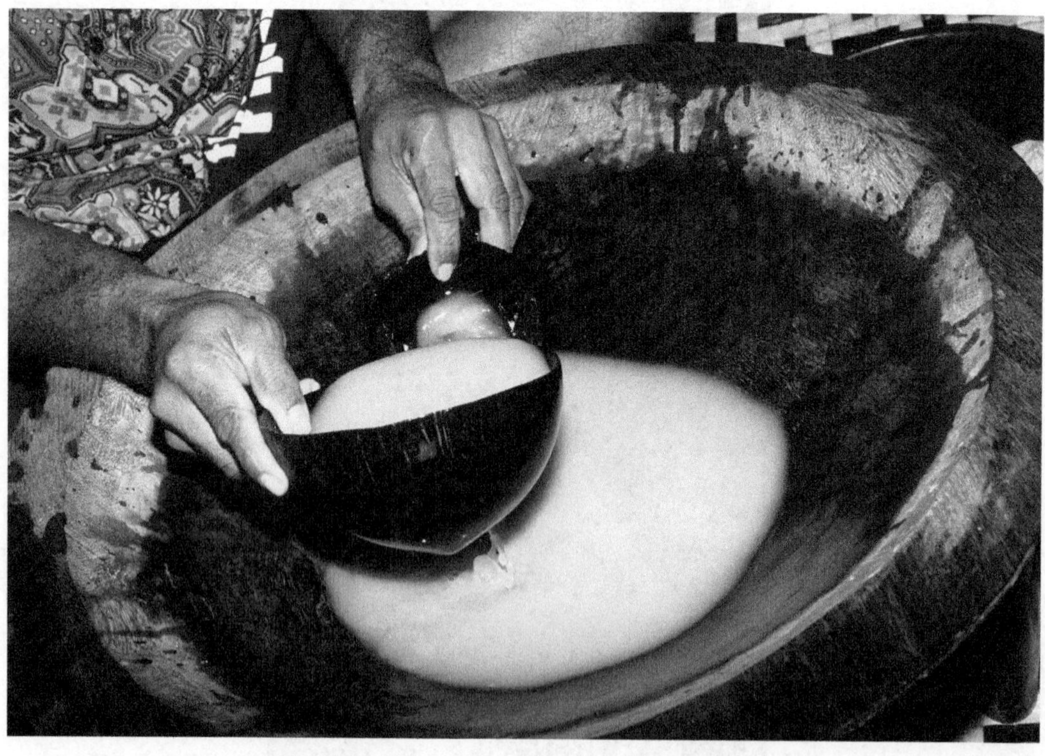

Caffeine is a legal natural drug that is widely used. Many people don't even know they are using this addictive drug because it is found in so many drinks. Cola, coffee, tea and some other energy drinks contain high levels of caffeine. It gives a mild high and increases concentration. Caffeine keeps you awake and makes you feel like you have more energy. If you drink too much it can make you irritable. Caffeine is addictive and some people may suffer from withdrawal symptoms if they drink cola or coffee a lot.

The health effects of caffeine are not yet clear. However drinking lots of sugary energy drinks like cola greatly increase the risk of tooth decay, obesity and diabetes. Diabetes and heart disease are major health problems in Pacific countries.

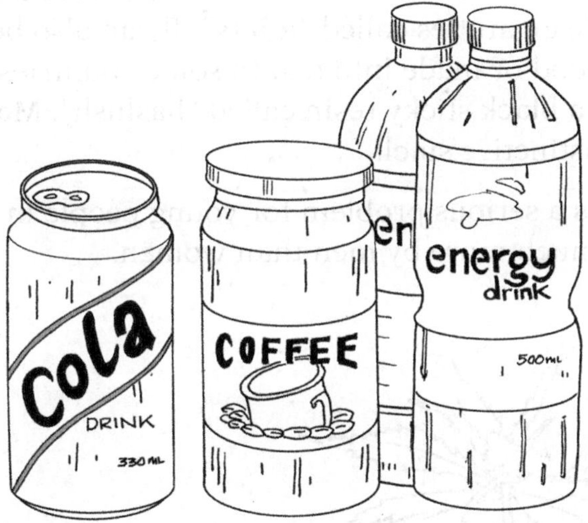

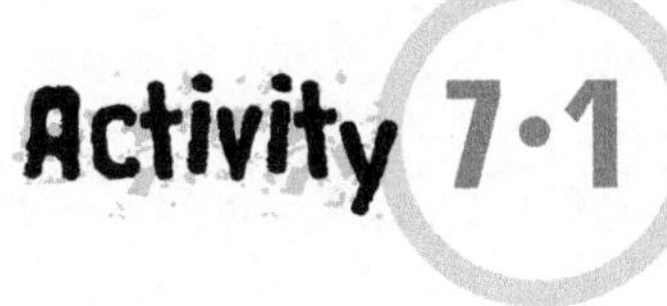

Work with a friend to try and rank legal drugs.

1 Which ones are the most dangerous to people's health?
2 Which ones are less dangerous?
3 Which legal drugs will you and your friends try to avoid? Why?

Chapter 8 Marijuana

Marijuana is an illegal drug that is widely available. It comes from the hemp plant (*Cannabis sativa*) that is common in PNG. Marijuana has many different names including "spak brus", "cannabis", "grass" and "weed".

Usually people smoke the dry shredded leaves, stems and seeds of the plant in homemade cigarettes called "joints". It can also be smoked in a pipe, mixed with food or made into tea. In some countries, marijuana is concentrated into a black sticky resin called "hashish". Marijuana smoke has a sweet and distinctive smell.

Marijuana abuse is a serious problem for young people in the Pacific region. It is used much more by men than women.

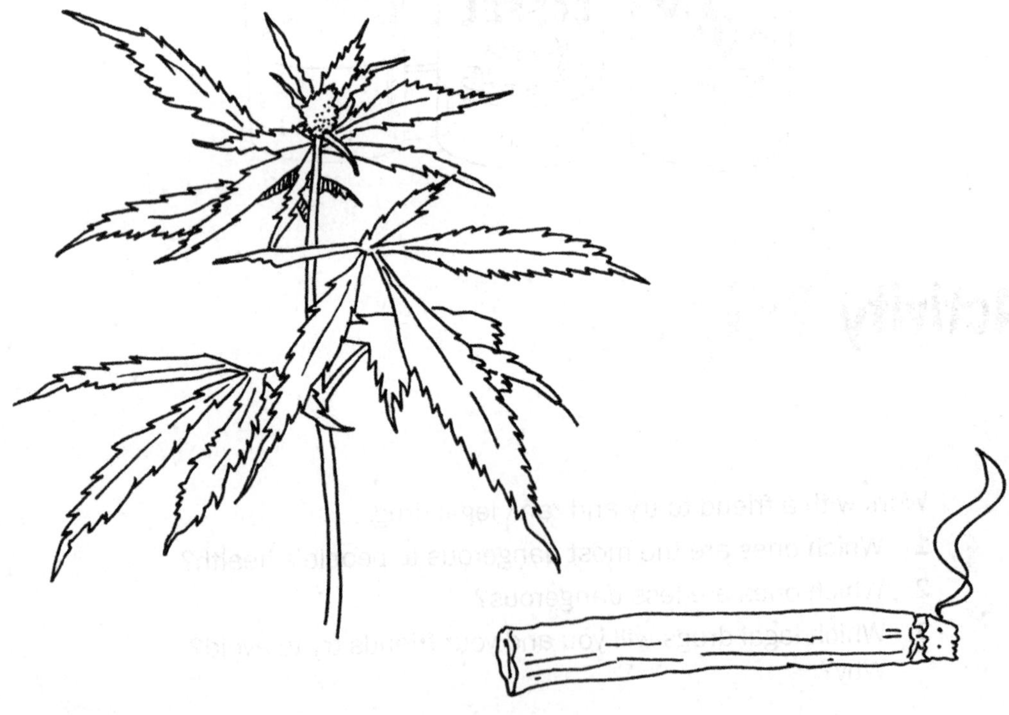

Facts about marijuana

- Marijuana contains many chemicals but the most powerful one is called THC (delta-9-tetrahydrocannabinol). This chemical is absorbed into the bloodstream and carried to all parts of the body.
- The effect on the person depends on the strength of the marijuana and how much is smoked.
- Sometimes people feel little or no effect from the drug. Sometimes people feel relaxed, energetic or dizzy. They might giggle and laugh a lot and be uncoordinated. Many people in PNG become aggressive after smoking marijuana.
- Sometimes people feel thirsty and hungry after smoking and they may feel worried and disorientated.
- Marijuana changes the way your mind works. This effect can last several hours if you smoke a lot or if the marijuana is strong. Several hours afterwards, most people feel very sleepy.

Laws about marijuana

- If you are caught growing, carrying or selling marijuana you will be expelled from school, or fined. You may be sent to prison for up to two years.
- In PNG, smoking marijuana can lead to bad behaviour or violence. This is different to many countries where marijuana is used for relaxation and chilling out.
- In PNG, this drug is often used with home-brew alcohol until the person is completely out of control.

The effects of marijuana:

- poor decision-making and loss of self-control which can lead to unprotected sex and other risky behaviour
- poor memory and lower reaction times
- lung cancer, blood clots and heart disease from smoke
- lack of interest in work or school
- addiction to the effects of the drug
- long-term damage to the brain and decision-making abilities
- getting into trouble with the police, school, family and community leaders.

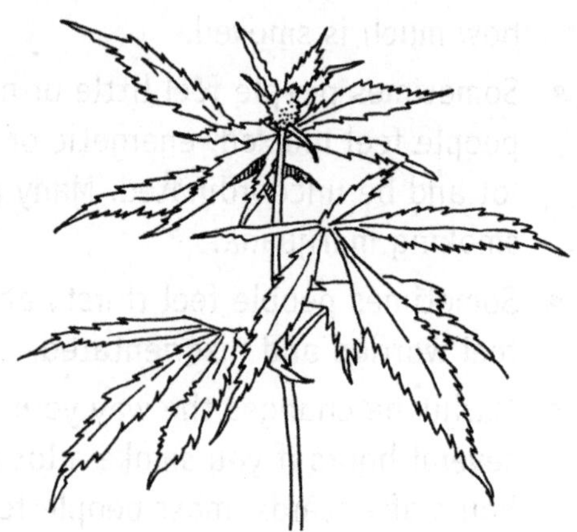

Activity 8·1

1. Write down three reasons why you would not use marijuana.
2. Now write down three goals in your life which smoking marijuana would affect – include a goal for the next six months, a goal for the next year, and a goal for the next five years.
3. Finally, use your goals and assertive language to write down what you would say if someone offered you marijuana to smoke.

The effects of marijuana on family and community

'When my brother started smoking spak brus with his gang, he stopped going to school and studying. He even stopped working in his garden. It was very sad and I miss him.' **Pita**

'We have had to ask for money from wantoks to pay my son's village court fine for being drunk and smoking marijuana. We felt a lot of shame.' **Miriam**

'My son used to have a small business making money from his garden. Now that money is wasted on alcohol and marijuana. He says that the drug gives him energy and confidence but I think he seems shy and confused now.' **Frank**

'I hear stories of young men with mental health problems from smoking. I worry about my grandson. What can we do?' **Elizabeth**

'I miss my brother. When he was on his own he was fun to play with. Now he is with this gang he scares me. You never know how they might behave.' **Simon**

'All my grandson's friends do is drink and smoke and expect rice to be on the table and school fees paid. This is not the right way to behave. Many of the women say they are scared of this group of youths.' **Maria**

Activity 8·2

What would you say to a peer or sibling if he or she said:

1. 'Marijuana doesn't harm anyone, does it?'
2. 'Smoking marijuana gives you energy, doesn't it?'
3. 'People drink alcohol. What is wrong with marijuana?'
4. 'I'll only smoke it once in a while. My friends won't pressure me.'

Sam's story

Sam is a fit and hardworking player in the village volleyball team. He works hard at school and has some ambitions for the future. Sam wants to follow in his mother's footsteps as a teacher. He doesn't drink much, but recently his mates have been sharing and smoking the marijuana that one of them is growing in the bush. Sam likes the effect it has on him. It makes him feel good. But it also makes him feel out of control and shy. Sam is not sure whether he should smoke again. His mates always seem to do something stupid when they smoke. Today is the big volleyball final. Sam's village should win. But as they walk to the next village, Sam's mate offers him a smoke. It is marijuana. What Sam decides to do next will affect his life forever ...

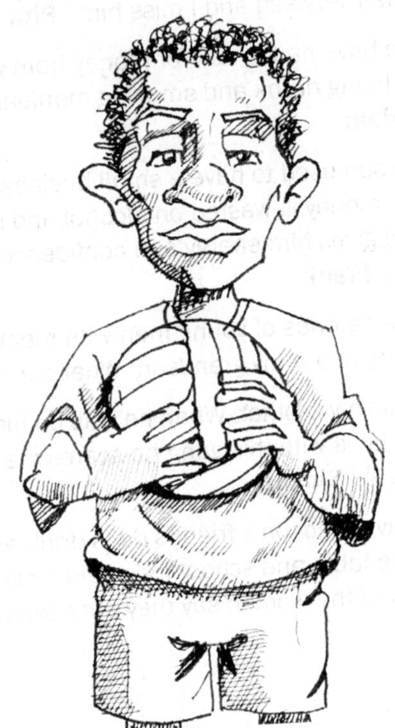

Activity 8·3

1 Write two different endings for Sam's story – what might happen if Sam takes the joint and what might happen if he doesn't?

2 For each story, write what the consequences might be for Sam in one year's time.

Chapter 9 Petrol, glue, aerosols and amphetamines

Petrol, glue and aerosols are also known as solvents. It is illegal to use these as drugs and it is rare for young people in PNG to abuse them. However, solvent abuse is a serious problem in other countries such as in Aboriginal communities in Australia and in the slums of big cities in the developing world.

Young people sniff the chemicals in petrol, spray cans and glue to get high. It makes them feel dizzy and out of control. These chemicals are very dangerous and poisonous. In the short term, they lead to painful headaches, changes in behaviour and loss of body functions. They can lead to brain and heart damage very quickly and can seriously affect your mental and physical ability. Sniffing petrol, paints and glue is very risky behaviour.

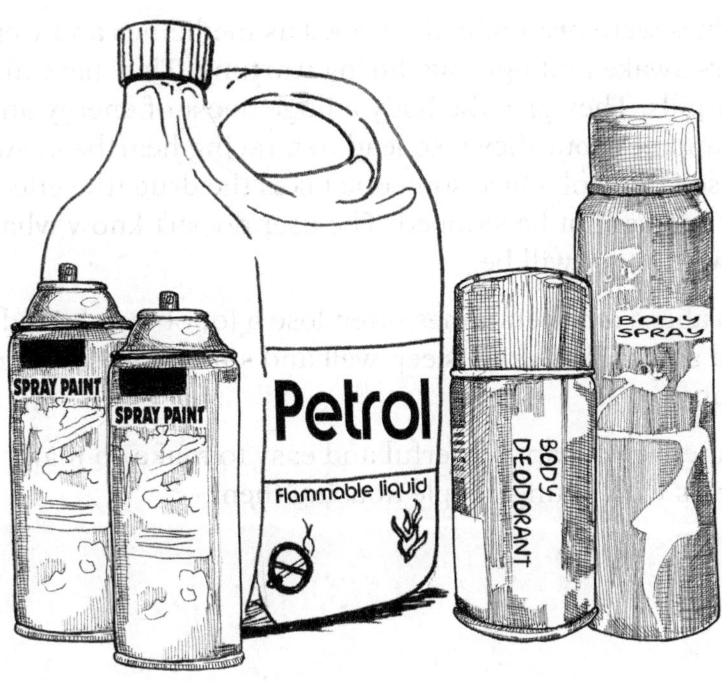

Amphetamines are illegal drugs that are common in countries surrounding the South Pacific but they are not common in PNG. They are powerful chemicals made in illegal laboratories and are usually sold as a powder to be snorted up the nose, swallowed or smoked. There are different types of amphetamines including 'ice', which is injected. This is extremely addictive and gives a powerful feeling of strength.

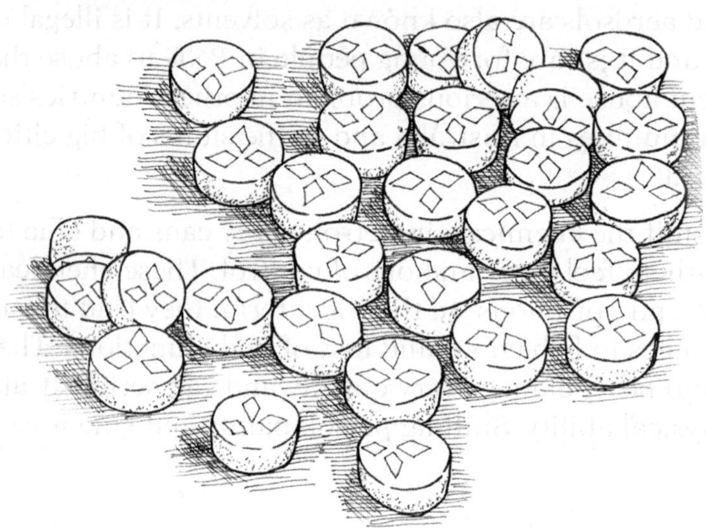

Amphetamines were originally developed as medicines and were used to keep soldiers awake and fighting during wartime. They have also been used as diet pills. They give the body a huge boost of energy and a strong feeling of happiness but they also lead to a racing heartbeat, sweating and loss of self-control. Once someone takes the drug, the effect can last a long time and cannot be stopped. The user doesn't know what is in the drug or how strong it will be.

People who abuse amphetamines often lose a lot of weight and have lots of spots and sores. They don't sleep well and suffer from paranoia and hallucinations.

Amphetamines are cheap, powerful and easy to make so many countries have problems with young people abusing them.

Chapter 10 Illegal drugs in other countries

There are many illegal drugs that are used by people in other countries. These drugs are rarely or never abused in PNG, but you will often hear about them in the international media.

 Ecstasy

This illegal drug gives the user a high, happy feeling and a sense of energy that lasts several hours. It is usually taken as a pill by people in nightclubs. But users do not know what other chemicals are mixed up in the pill, or how strong the pill will be, which can be dangerous.

Ecstasy raises the heart rate and can cause mild hallucinations and loss of focus and memory. It also changes the body's systems and there is a risk of dehydration or drinking too much water. It is risky to mix ecstasy with alcohol. Long-term effects include mild depression.

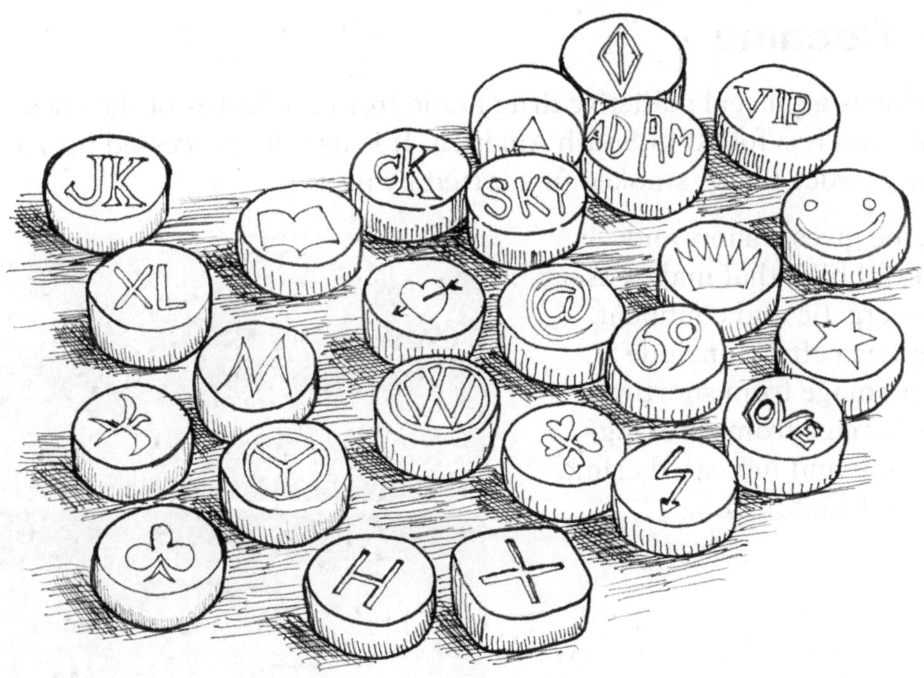

Heroin

Heroin is extracted from the poppy flower. It is a powerful illegal drug that can be made into painkillers. People who abuse heroin usually smoke it or inject it.

Heroin causes a short-term but very powerful high. People who abuse heroin say that using it helps them escape from the stress of daily life. Heroin is extremely addictive. Once someone is addicted to heroin it is very difficult to give up.

The side effects include a risk of death by overdosing, a risk of contracting HIV/AIDS and hepatitis from sharing dirty or used needles, and damage to the brain and body from the drug. Users build up a tolerance to heroin – this means they need to take more and more of the drug to get a high. This leads to a lot of crime as users steal to buy more drugs.

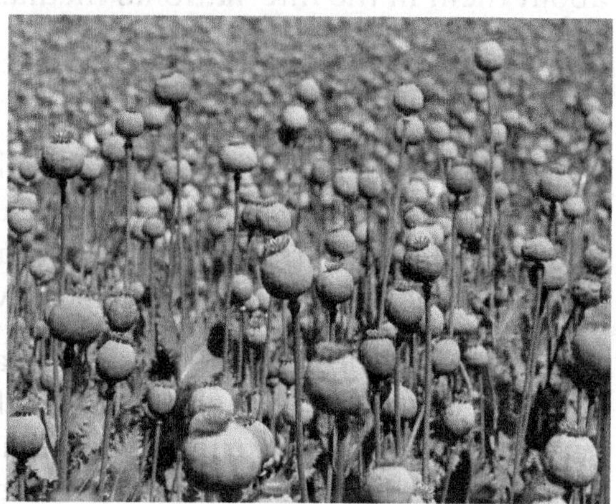

Cocaine

Cocaine is an illegal addictive drug made from the leaves of the coca plant, which is found in South America. It is usually processed into a fine white powder that is smoked or snorted by users.

Cocaine gives a short and powerful high that makes users feel energetic and confident. Long-term effects include nose damage from snorting, lung damage from smoking, addiction and increased crime to feed the addiction.

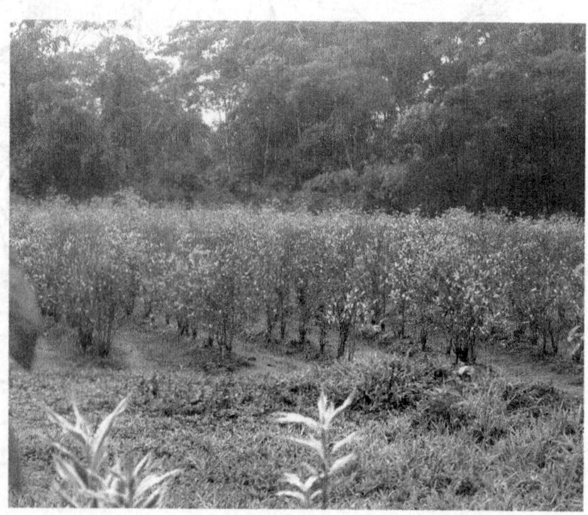

LSD

This is a manufactured chemical that has extremely powerful effects on the mind. It is usually taken as a small dot of the LSD chemical (lysergic acid diethylamide) on paper, so judging the strength of the drug is difficult.

Users have hallucinations and out-of-body experiences and can experience anxiety. LSD changes the way they see, hear and feel – sound, colours and objects appear to change. Each "trip" lasts several hours and users cannot sleep during this time. The mental effects of LSD can be risky because decision-making skills are affected. The long-term effects are not known but are likely to include mental health issues.

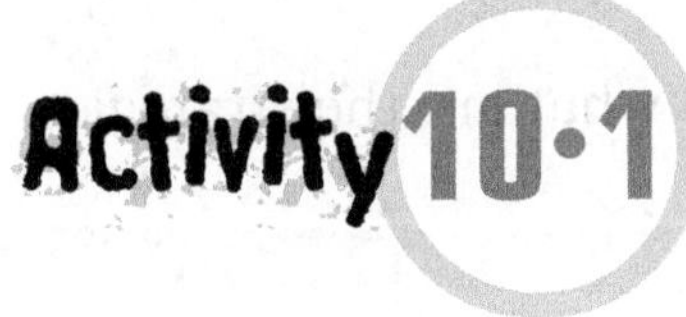

1. With a partner, try to rank these illegal drugs in order of how risky they are to people's health.
2. Which ones are the most dangerous to the individual?
3. Which ones are most damaging to the community?

Chapter 11 Resisting drugs and alcohol

Most young people in PNG are introduced to both legal and illegal drugs by friends. It is a tradition in our culture to share with friends, family and wantoks. This can put pressure on young people to use drugs and alcohol.

You don't need to use drugs and alcohol even if everyone else is doing it. You might want to keep control over your mind, your emotions and your health. It is not easy to resist using drugs if they are common in your community, but many people do.

Making wise decisions is an important life skill. So what are the strategies for resisting pressure to use drugs and alcohol?

Feeling good about yourself

'I don't need to drink or smoke to feel like a bikman. I am a happy and cheerful person and I feel confident about my decisions. I also keep myself busy – rugby touch, volleyball and my studies. I want to be a good role model for my younger sisters.'

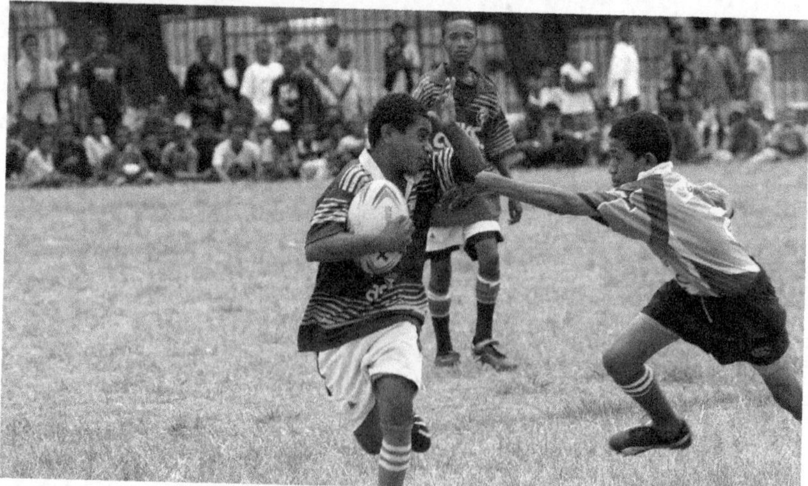

Learn to say 'no thanks'

Being assertive and clear in terms of what you will and won't do is very important. If you don't want to risk your health, you need to learn how to say "no".

Choose your friends carefully

A good friend won't put you under pressure to risk your health or make you do something you don't feel happy about. You should be a good friend too – never pressure someone into drinking or smoking.

'I used to hang around after school with a group of friends. They started drinking home-brew and got into fights. We were all expected to drink but I could see what would eventually happen. It was hard to leave them but I made excuses and found some new friends through Church. I miss the old friends but I couldn't risk it.'

Learn about the risks

Find out how legal and illegal drugs affect you and your body. Make a wise decision and stick to it.

Learn from your mistakes

Everyone makes mistakes and no one is perfect. But a smart person learns from their mistakes and tries to improve their life.

Learn from your role models

Role models are very important. How do they cope with the pressure to use drugs? What lessons have they learnt? Remember you are a role model for your peers and your younger brothers, sisters, cousins and schoolmates.

Watch out for risky situations

There are many times when you will be under pressure to do something that might risk your health or your safety. Learn to avoid these situations and try to leave if you think you might be at risk.

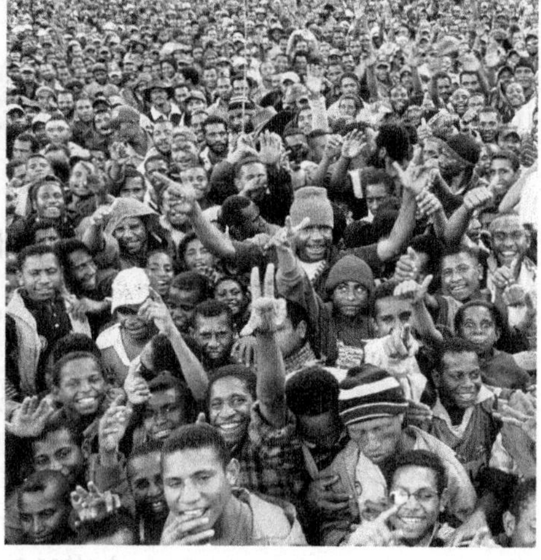

Activity 11·1

Mark's friends are making home-brew in the school dormitory. One night he is sitting with his mates when they start to hand around a cordial bottle full of home-brew. Mark doesn't want to share.

1. What would you do and what would you say if you were Mark? Try to think of assertive ways to say "no".
2. What do you think would happen next?
3. What are the choices for Mark? Sort these into the best and worst strategies.

Activity 11·2

1. With a group of peers, list risky times and places for drug and alcohol abuse in your age group.
2. Draw a map of your community and label the risky places. Why are they risky? At what times? (For example, places where home-brew is sold, harvest time, dances and sporting events.)

Chapter 12 Giving up drugs and alcohol

It is important to remember that many people start using drugs when they are young. The best way to avoid getting addicted is not to use them in the first place, but many people do drink, do smoke and some do use illegal drugs. The challenge is to give it up! This can be difficult because the body gets used to the drug and craves it when it doesn't have it.

It is important to be able to see the signs of drug and alcohol abuse in your friends and relatives. You might be able to help them give up drugs and improve their health. That is how a good friend behaves. Some of the warning signs of drug and alcohol abuse could be:

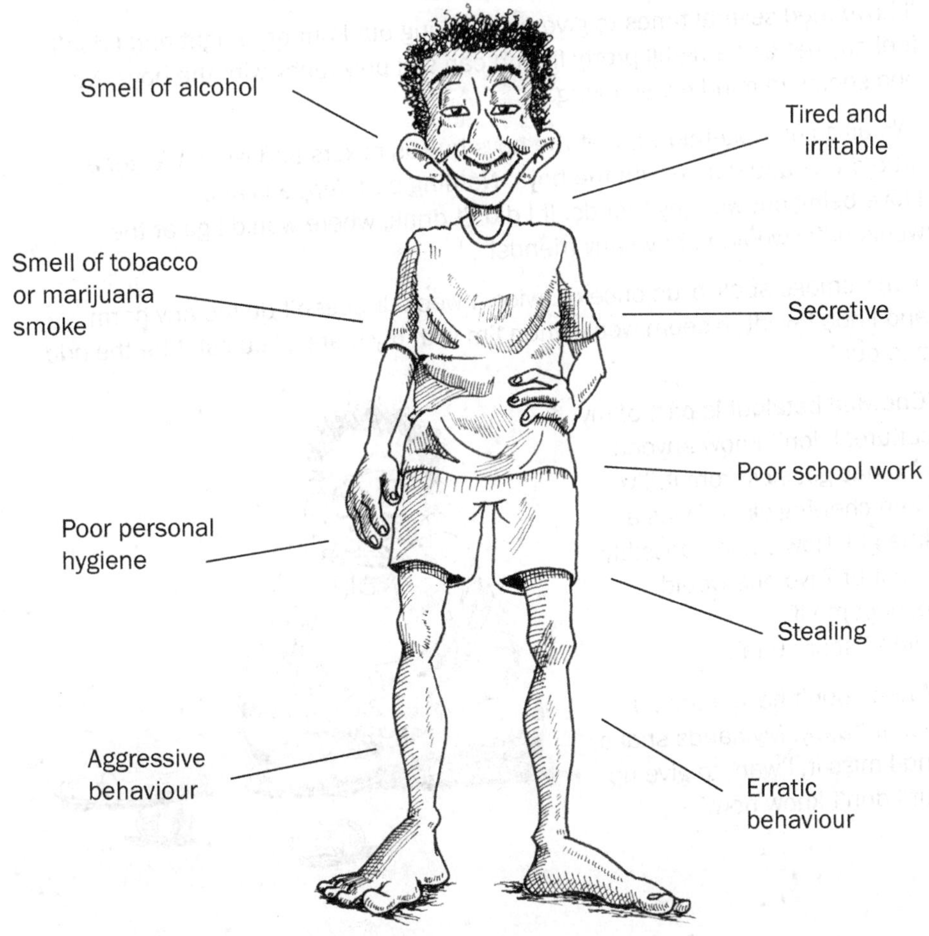

Activity 12·1

- Why is it hard to give up drugs like tobacco, alcohol or marijuana? List the reasons and sort them into physical, emotional and social reasons.
- Which drugs do you think would be hardest to give up? Why?

Why do people find it hard to give up drugs and alcohol?

'I have tried several times to give up smoking but I put on weight and I don't feel any better. I am still pretty fit and can still play rugby with the boys. No one seems to mind my smoking.'

'We all go out together and let the boys buy us mixers and wine. We get a little drunk and dance with the boys. Nothing bad happens and I love being out with my friends. If I didn't drink, where would I go at the weekend? I wouldn't have any friends!'

'I only smoke spak brus once or twice a week. It doesn't do me any harm and I don't want to seem weak when I'm with my mates. You can't be the odd one out.'

'Chewing betelnut is part of my culture. I don't know anyone who has got sick from it. I've been chewing since I was a little girl. How could I possibly give it up? No one would respect me if I didn't share buai.'

'When I don't have a drink I feel unhappy. My hands shake and I miss it. I want to give up but I don't know how.'

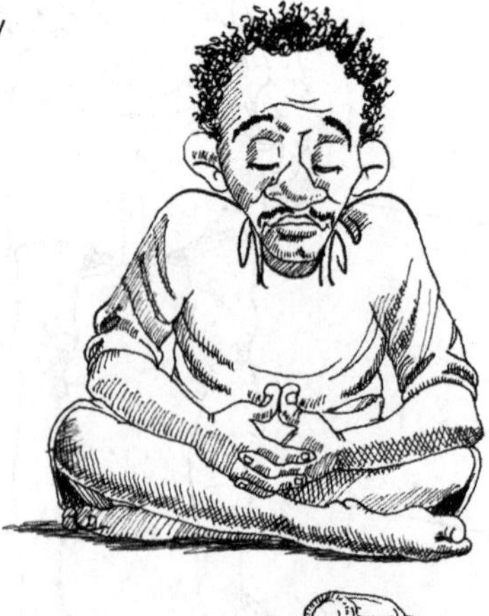
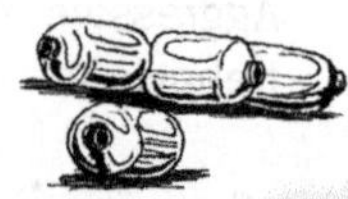

The most important reason to give up drug and alcohol use is your health. Almost all drugs damage your body in some way and most of this damage can be reversed if you give up. If you help a family member to quit drinking or smoking, you are doing a good thing.

 Ten-step plan to quit

1. Recognise you have a problem

Young people naturally think they will live a long time and some of the health effects from drug and alcohol abuse may take many years to show up. So the first step is realising you have a problem with drugs or alcohol and that you want to do something about it.

There are two ways of quitting something:

- Reduce the use – slowly and steadily reduce the number of times you use the drug.
- Abstinence – stop using the drug immediately and completely (counsellors sometimes call this 'cold turkey').

2. Educate yourself

Find out about the dangers of drug and alcohol abuse. Find out who can help you and what you will need to do about quitting. Speak to other people who have given up the drug and learn how they quit. Learn about any withdrawal symptoms, such as headaches or shaking, and how to deal with these.

3. Make a plan of action

Plan how you are going to reduce the use of or abstain from using the drug. For example, if you are a heavy chewer, you might plan to only chew betelnut twice a day for a month and then once a day after that.

You can set yourself rules and an allowance to help you decide how to reduce your addiction. You should also plan for times and places. For example, if you always drink home-brew on a sports tour, you can change club or stay with family friends rather than with the rest of the team.

4. Set yourself a realistic target

This step is very important. Set a target and a time you can achieve.

- 'I'll only take enough money to the club for two bottles of beer.'
- 'I will quit chewing by Easter.'
- 'I will halve the number of cigarettes I smoke in a week.'

5. Find a healthy substitute

A lot of drug abuse is the result of unhealthy habits. A lot of people smoke or chew more when they drink alcohol. Smokers get used to having a cigarette in their hands. Chewers get used to having *buai* or *daka* to share with friends during lunchtime. Make sure you replace an unhealthy habit with a healthy one.

- 'I will keep sugar-free chewing gum in my pockets for when I want a smoke.'
- 'I am going to drink juice or a bottle of water between each bottle of beer.'
- 'Each week I am going to deposit the money I save on smokes in the local microfinance bank.'
- 'At the end of the game, I will eat bananas and pineapple from my sports bag rather than have a smoke and a coke.'

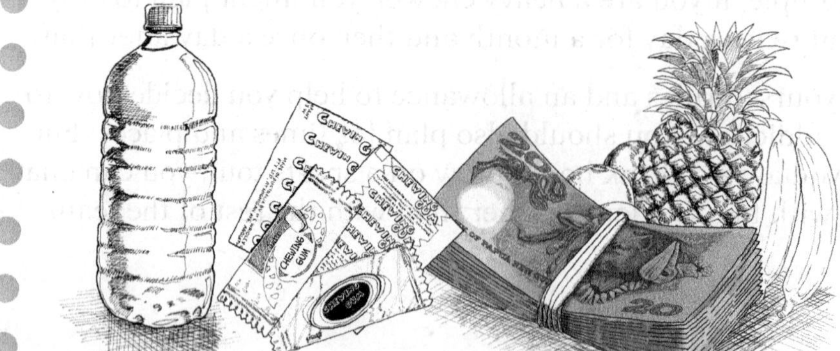

6. Avoid temptation

You should also think carefully about *when* and *where* and *with who* you use the drug you want to give up. If you always smoke and drink with a certain group of friends or at a certain time of the week, what can you do to reduce the peer pressure?

- 'I will give up going to the bush nightclub and join a sports club.'
- 'Instead of hanging around chewing and talking, I am going to work my garden and make some money.'
- 'When I walk to school with Christine she always offers me a smoke, so I will walk with my younger sisters instead.'
- 'I chew when I get bored so I will keep a good book in my bilum.'
- 'When we go off to hunt in the bush, we always end up drinking home-brew. I am going to start a chicken project instead.'

7. Ask for help

Giving up an addictive drug on your own can be very difficult. There are lots of people who can help you and mentor you, such as:

- older brothers and sisters
- good friends
- family members
- your local pastor
- an understanding teacher
- a boyfriend or girlfriend
- a health worker
- a community organisation, NGO or counselling group.

Explain to them what your target is and ask them for help with your plan. Report your progress to them and ask for their support and advice if things are tough.

If you always end up drinking or smoking or chewing with friends, tell them why you are giving up and tell them not to offer you anything or put you under pressure. If they put you under pressure to use drugs and alcohol then you should really think about whether these are good friends to have. You have a choice to be part of their group and your health should be important to you.

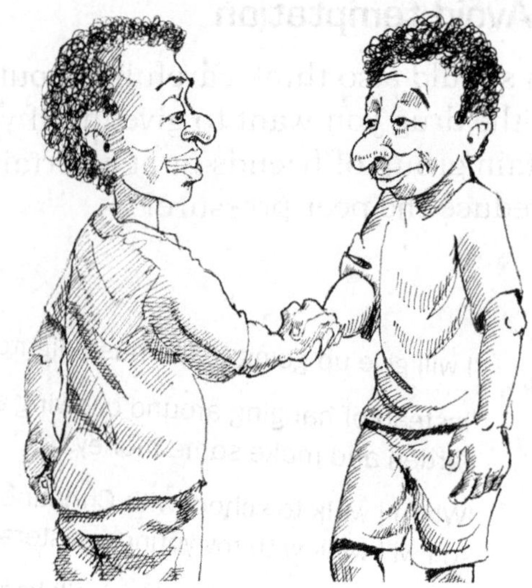

Practise being assertive and what you are going to say when someone offers you drugs or alcohol.

- 'No thanks, I want white teeth for kissing and smiling.'
- 'Thanks for not offering one to me. I'm trying to give up and get healthy.'
- 'Thanks but no thanks. Here, have some gum.'
- 'I haven't drunk any home-brew for two months thanks to you.'
- 'Sorry, I don't have any. I am quitting. I have some peanuts in my bag though if you want one.'
- 'No way, bro. You told me you were giving up.'

8. Supporting others

It is much easier to give up drugs and alcohol if you have someone to help you. It is also important for you to help and support your own friends and family to give up. If you have a health issue you want to improve, perhaps there are other friends who also have the same problem. Support your friends and family if they want to give up.

9. Monitor your progress

This is very important and good for your self-esteem. There are many ways of keeping track of your progress, such as:

- a diary
- a wall chart
- weekly meetings with a supportive friend
- a jar to keep the coins you would usually spend on *buai* or smokes.

In this way you can keep track of your progress towards quitting and becoming healthier.

Since giving up buai I have saved:

Week 1	K4.50
Week 2	K4.50
Week 3	K4.50
Week 4	
Week 5	

Running total: K13.50

10. Don't give up trying to quit

It can be hard to give up some drugs. They can be very addictive or they could be common in your social circle. If your plan doesn't work, don't give up. Keep trying. For example, it takes people two to three times on average to give up smoking tobacco.

Look at Annette's personal action plan for giving up smoking. Now select one thing that you want to give up or reduce to improve your health and write a personal action plan of your own.

ANNETTE'S HEALTH – PERSONAL ACTION PLAN

What is the health problem?	Why do I want to give up?	What is my plan for giving up?	What is my target?	Who can help me quit?
I smoke bought and hand-rolled cigarettes after volleyball, and when I walk into town with my friends. I smoke and share two to four cigarettes a day.	1. My younger brother might copy me. 2. My clothes and breath smell. 3. I am worried about getting cancer and not being fit enough for the volleyball team. 4. I want to save money.	1. Chew gum and have a sports drink after volleyball. 2. Take one drag on the cigarette and pass it on. 3. Tell my team and my friends that I am trying to quit. 4. Ask my younger brother if he can smell smoke on my clothes. 5. Reduce my smoking to one cigarette a day over the next three weeks.	Stop smoking after three weeks.	• Friends • Brothers and sisters • Sports coach and team-mates

MY HEALTH – PERSONAL ACTION PLAN

Name: ______________________________

Village: ______________________________

Age: ______________________________

What is the health problem?	Why do I want to give up?	What is my plan for giving up?	What is my target?	Who can help me quit?

Organisations that can help

There may be organisations in your local area that can help you give up or reduce your drug and alcohol use. There are non-governmental organisations (NGOs) and government services that work with young people. Your school can also help through Health and Personal Development subjects and school-based counsellors.

Many schools are health-promoting schools that have strict rules on smoking and drinking. Students should get involved in their school to make it a healthy environment. Is your school a health-promoting school?

Activity 12·4

Research who could help people give up drugs and alcohol in your local community or town. Ask at the school, your church and the health centre. Try looking in the telephone book to see if there are any national organisations and help lines. Make a list of these organisations.

Activity 12·5

With three peers, plan and conduct an awareness plan for your local community for one drug of addiction. You could use posters, leaflets, talks in the market, drama and songs, write persuasive letters to community leaders, or make a notice board. You can also try peer education – speak to your friends about how to say "no" to drugs and alcohol and how to resist peer pressure and stay healthy.

Chapter 13 HIV/AIDS

HIV/AIDS, sexually transmitted infections (STIs) and unplanned pregnancy are serious issues for young women and men. Drugs and alcohol abuse increase the risk of being infected with HIV or STIs or having an unplanned pregnancy.

Alcohol and marijuana abuse are major causes of rape and violence. Eighty per cent of rape victims report that drugs or alcohol were involved in the attack. Sixty per cent of victims said that the rapist had been drinking alcohol. The true number could be higher. Alcohol and marijuana abuse are major causes of rape, violence and HIV and STI infection in PNG. It is a problem the whole community and all young people must do something about. Being drunk or high puts *you* at risk.

If young people are drunk or high on drugs they might make poor decisions.

- A young woman might put herself at risk of being raped or attacked.
- A young man might rape or attack someone.
- They might have sex without a condom and be infected with HIV or STIs.
- A young woman might get pregnant.
- A young man might decide to have sex with a sex worker.
- They might get robbed.
- They could be persuaded to do something risky.
- They could get involved in an argument and violence.
- They will take risks and do things they might regret the next day.

Summary of drugs of addiction

Drug	Legal or illegal?	Health effects	Social impacts
Alcohol	Beer, wine, spirits – legal Home-brew – illegal	• Intoxication • Hangover • Serious behaviour problems and violence • Abuse and binge-drinking leads to cirrhosis of the liver, heart disease, obesity	• Money generated or money wasted • Abuse leads to violence, rape, infection with HIV and STIs, family breakdown, community disturbance • Lost productivity due to violence and ill health
Tobacco	Manufactured or home-grown – legal	• Nicotine addiction • Stained teeth and fingers • Lung, mouth and throat cancer, heart disease • Second-hand smoke harms others	• Money generated or money wasted • Increased medical costs to country and family • Lost productivity due to violence and ill health
Betelnut	Legal	• Mild high • Lack of appetite • Stained teeth and clothes • Mouth cancer	• Money generated or money wasted • Litter and stained environment • Increased risk of tuberculosis • Lost productivity due to violence and ill health

Drug	Legal or illegal?	Health effects	Social impacts
Kava	Legal	• Mild high • Possible liver damage • Scaly skin • Nausea	• Money generated or money wasted
Caffeine	Legal	• Increased energy and concentration • Hard to sleep • Sugary drinks lead to tooth decay, obesity, diabetes and heart attacks	• Increased medical costs from obesity and diabetes
Marijuana	Illegal	• Lung damage and lung cancer • Lack of concentration • Increased risk of mental health problems • Possibility of hallucinations and paranoia	• Social problems and poor behaviour • Can lead to aggression and violence • Money generated or money wasted • Lost productivity due to violence and ill health
Solvents (glue, petrol, aerosols)	Illegal	• Headaches • Bad skin • Risk of sudden death	• Social and school problems • Family break-ups

Drug	Legal or illegal?	Health effects	Social impacts
Amphetamines (speed)	Illegal	• Energy and a feeling of happiness and power • Reduced appetite and heart rate • Hallucinations, aggression, paranoia, weight loss and poor sleeping	• Health and social problems • Violence and crime
Methamphetamine (ice)	Illegal	• Same as for amphetamines • Health risks of injecting and smoking including dangers of sharing needles • Addiction	• Violence, serious health problems, very short life expectancy for addicts • Serious social problems
Ecstasy	Illegal	• Energy and intense happiness • Sleeplessness • Mild hallucinations • Unknown chemicals in the pill • Risk of dehydration, over-heating or drinking too much water	• Mild depression for heavy users • Risk of death for users who take it when dancing or mixing ecstasy with alcohol

Drug	Legal or illegal?	Health effects	Social impacts
Heroin	Illegal	• Powerfully addictive, strong high and no feeling of pain or anxiety • Risk of HIV/AIDS and other diseases from unclean needles	• Severe addiction and ill heath • Overdosing leads to death • Crime and robbery for addicts to feed their habit
Cocaine	Illegal	• Feeling of power and energy • Depression when the drug wears off • Addictive (especially crack cocaine) • Heart and nose damage	• Severe addiction and illness • Crime and robbery for addicts to feed their habit
LSD	Illegal	• Strong hallucinations	• Mental health problems from users when on the drug

More information about drugs and alcohol

Smoking

www.quitnow.info.au

Drug abuse

www.drugs-info.co.uk

PNG National Narcotics Bureau

Alcohol

www.alcohol.gov.au

Your local health centre or hospital will be able to give you more information on drug and alcohol services in your area.

Counselling services in PNG

PNG Department of Education Guidance Branch

Many Provinces have Guidance Officers and most secondary schools have school-based counsellors.

Catholic Family Services 325 9917

Lifeline Hotline 326 0011

Peer education and youth NGOs

Save the Children

Anglicare StopAIDS

Department of Education Population Education

UNICEF

Glossary

addiction
when your body needs to have a drug or you feel ill

assertiveness
saying what you want without being weak or aggressive. This is an important life skill.

binge drinking
when someone drinks too much alcohol at one time. For example, "six-to-six" drinking is when men drink all night with friends. Binge-drinking is dangerous to your health and leads to poor behaviour.

black market medicines
illegal selling of medicine stolen from Government health centres and stores

bronchitis
swelling of the tubes in the lungs, which causes coughing, lots of phlegm and shortness of breath. This condition is caused by tobacco and marijuana smoke.

cancer
a dangerous growth or tumour that grows inside the body. Some cancers can be caused by poisons and chemicals and can be fatal.

carbon monoxide
poisonous gas breathed in by smokers

cirrhosis
liver damage caused by alcohol abuse

drug
a substance that changes the body physically, mentally or emotionally

emphysema
extreme shortness of breath and feeling of suffocation. This condition results from lung damage caused by tobacco smoke and can lead to death.

ethanol
the chemical name for alcohol

health
the physical, mental and emotional state of a person

high
a feeling of energy or unusual physical feelings, and an altered physical, emotional or mental state

illegal
something that is against the law

LSD
the active chemical in LSD (acid) called lysergic acid diethylamide

medicine
a legal drug, which treats a sickness or illness

nicotine
the addictive chemical found in tobacco smoke

non-prescription medicines
legal medicines that can be bought in a pharmacy or supermarket without a prescription from a doctor, including Panadol and cough medicines

overdose
poisoning caused by taking too much of a drug which can lead to death

passive smoking
when someone breathes in someone else's smoke. This is very harmful and can lead to lung cancer, asthma and other illnesses.

peer pressure
when a person's friends and peers persuade them to do something or a person does what their friends do to be part of a group. This behaviour can be negative or positive.

prescription medicines
legal medicines that you can only get with a prescription from a doctor or health worker

resisting pressure
saying "no" to peer pressure to engage in risky behaviours such as smoking

second-hand smoke
see passive smoking

side effects
possible problems caused by medicines or drugs such as upset stomach, bad skin or nausea

smoker's cough
a dry persistent cough as the body tries to cough up tar and other damage from smoking, caused by damage to the lung tubes

THC
the active chemical in marijuana (delta-9-tetrahydrocannabinol)

units
the measurement for alcohol. One bottle of beer is around 1½ units.